# Skin Cancer - Past, Present and Future

*Edited by Gerardo Cazzato and Giuseppe Ingravallo*

Published in London, United Kingdom

Skin Cancer - Past, Present and Future
http://dx.doi.org/10.5772/intechopen.111249
Edited by Gerardo Cazzato and Giuseppe Ingravallo

Contributors
Adeeb Shehzad, Anna Jghamadze, Anne Callahan, Catherine Shachaf, Csongor Németh, Eter Natelauri, Farhan Hameed, Francesco Fortarezza, Gerardo Cazzato, Giuseppe Ingravallo, Jenan Al-Matouq, Jie Xu, Jinhui Wang, Lele Lin, Muhammad Ammad Jamil, Muhammad Salman Khalid, Qiaochu Zhou, Rolland Gyulai, Serena Federico, Shan Zhang, Somia Mazhar, Yanan Zhang, Yoav Litvin, Zsuzsanna Lengyel



First published in London, United Kingdom, 2025 by IntechOpen
IntechOpen is the global imprint of INTECHOPEN LIMITED, registered in England and Wales, registration number: 11086078, 167-169 Great Portland Street, London, W1W 5PF, United Kingdom

For EU product safety concerns: IN TECH d.o.o., Prolaz Marije Krucifikse Kozulić 3, 51000 Rijeka, Croatia, info@intechopen.com or visit our website at intechopen.com.

British Library Cataloguing-in-Publication Data
A catalogue record for this book is available from the British Library

Skin Cancer - Past, Present and Future
Edited by Gerardo Cazzato and Giuseppe Ingravallo
p. cm.
Print ISBN 978-0-85466-827-4
Online ISBN 978-0-85466-826-7
eBook (PDF) ISBN 978-0-85466-828-1

# Meet the editor

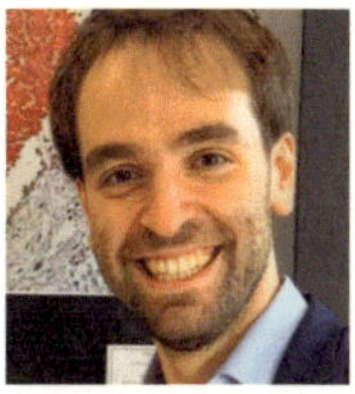

Gerardo Cazzato is an ICDP/UEMS Board Certified Dermatopathologist. He obtained a master's degree in medicine from the University of Bari "Aldo Moro" in Italy and a Ph.D. in clinical medicine, public health, and oncology at the same university. He is an International Fellow of the College of American Pathologists (IFCAP), and currently, he is an MSc Student of Molecular Pathology at the University of Cote d'Azur in France. Dr. Cazzato works as a pathologist at the University of Bari "Aldo Moro", particularly in Dermatopathology, Soft Tissue pathology and Bone pathology and has international research collaborations with different institutions. Dr. Cazzato has submitted more than 40 abstracts to international conferences, published more than 200 papers in peer-reviewed journals and authored six book chapters.

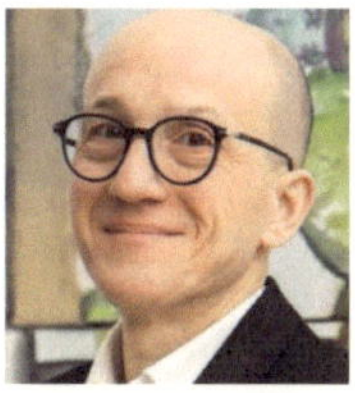

Giuseppe Ingravallo is a full professor of Pathology at the University of Bari "Aldo Moro" in Italy. He obtained his Ph.D. and a master's degree in medicine from the same University and worked in gastrointestinal pathology at the University of Padua in Italy. He is currently the director of the complex unit of pathological anatomy at the same hospital, specialising in hematopathology, neuropathology, skin pathology, and gastrointestinal pathology. He has won several Italian national research grants and collaborates with prestigious international institutions. He is the author of more than 300 papers and several book chapters and has contributed over 60 abstracts to international conferences.

# Contents

# Preface

Skin cancer (SC) represents one of the greatest medical challenges, both in terms of its diffusion and its ability to lead to death in a certain number of cases. Traditionally, SC has been divided into Melanoma and Non Melanoma Skin Cancer (NMSC), the latter group consisting of basal cell carcinoma (BCC), squamous cell carcinoma (SCC) and Merkel cell carcinoma (MCC). Moreover, with the refinement of molecular diagnostic methodologies, more and more findings are shedding light on the oncogenesis pathways responsible for the biology and behaviour of these neoplasms. Despite this, to date, still on the threshold of 2025, the histopathological diagnosis represents the Gold Standard of the correct diagnostic approach on which the beginning of the therapeutic and care pathway of the patient with SC is based. It is also important to emphasize that alongside surgical therapies, which continue to play a role of primary importance, research today is making it possible to discover new oncological therapies that can assist or, in some cases, replace the traditional surgical approach.

This first part of the publishing project 'Skin Cancer: Past, Present and Future' has gathered some significant contributions from authors from different regions of the globe, all of whom share the study of SC from different perspectives.

In particular, the first section, entitled 'Generalities and Epidemiology', focuses on a general discussion of SC with special attention to the epidemiological data of the different types updated to 2024. Section 2, titled 'Basal Cell Carcinoma (BCC)', provides an up-to-date review of basal cell carcinoma and multiple basal cell carcinoma syndromes, considering the most up-to-date molecular findings. Section 3, titled 'Alternative Therapy for BCC', is related to the possibility of using radiation therapy and topical Fluorouracil therapy for BCC, adding other possibilities to the therapeutic arsenal we have at our disposal. Finally, in section 4, titled 'Future Perspectives', the authors present a useful diagnostic imaging technique for biological activity to diagnose melanoma in its early phases.

As editors, we would like to publicly thank the authors, reviewers and all those who played an important role in making it possible to publish this book.

A special dedication goes to our teachers, now ascended into Heaven, to whom we owe so much, perhaps everything, of what we are and do.

**Dr. Gerardo Cazzato and Dr. Giuseppe Ingravallo**
Section of Molecular Pathology,
Department of Precision and Regenerative Medicine and Ionian Area (DiMePRe-J),
University of Bari "Aldo Moro",
Bari, Italy

Section 1

# Generalities and Epidemiology

Chapter 1

# Advances in Skin Cancer

*Jenan Al-Matouq*


## Abstract

Skin cancer has been associated with excessive sun exposure ever since the nineteenth century. The most common affected skin cells upon recurrent exposure to the sun include the squamous cells, basal cells, and Merkel cells. Basal cell carcinoma has the highest prevalence among the other types of skin cancer, but rarely metastasizes and is highly treatable. Squamous cell carcinoma, if left untreated, is inclined to penetrate the epidermis, invade into the dermis, and metastasize to other organs. Melanoma, however, is highly aggressive and has the least survival rates. Cumulative exposure to ultraviolet radiation mainly from the sun results in DNA damage, oxidative stress, inflammatory response, and gene mutations, all leading to the development of skin cancer. Many molecular pathways are affected by the mutations and can activate oncogenes, inactivate tumor suppressor genes, or impair DNA repair genes. This consequently can lead to increased proliferation, blood vessel growth, tumor invasion, evasion of immune response, and ultimately, metastasis. Early detection is vital to prevent cancer promotion and is mainly *via* histopathological techniques. Treatment options include surgical removal as the first-line treatment for early stages of skin cancer and immune therapy. An alternative emerging approach in the treatment of metastasized skin cancer is through nanotechnology that operates at a nanoscale increasing drug delivery and distribution in the body.


**Keywords:** epidermis, UV radiation, squamous cell carcinoma, basal cell carcinoma, melanoma

## 1. Introduction

### 1.1 Anatomy and histology of normal human skin

The layers of the skin include the superficial epidermis layer underlaid by a basement membrane separating it from the dermis layer, which in turn rests on the deepest layer called the hypodermis. The subcutaneous loose tissue and fat within the hypodermis support the skin and insulate body temperature [1].

The dermis layer is the thickest layer of the skin, which comprises hair follicles, sweat glands, blood vessels, and nerves that are held in place by collagen [1]. It also comprises fibroblasts, which are responsible for the synthesis of the extracellular matrix protein, collagen, elastin, and proteoglycan. Together, these patterns provide the skin with elasticity and strength. Immune cells such as lymphocytes and macrophages are also located in the dermis and help protect the body from foreign material (**Figure 1**) [3].

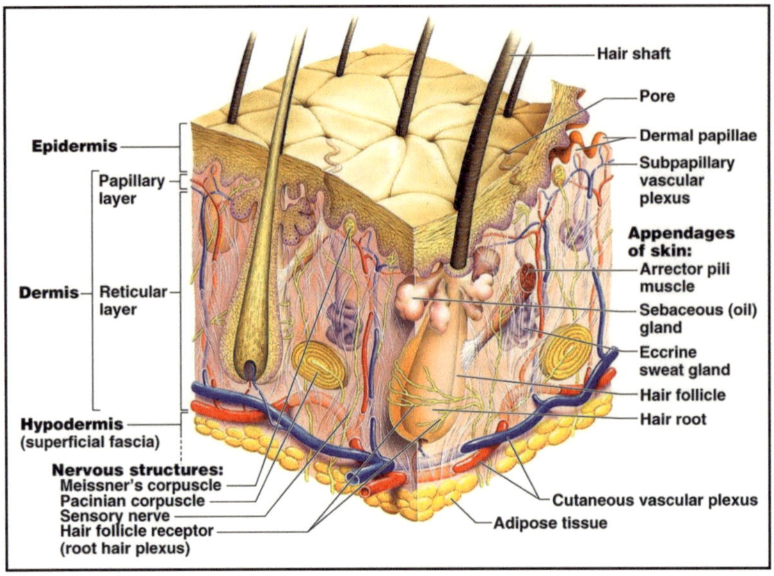


**Figure 1.**
*The structural features of the skin (Copyright @ 2007 Pearson Education, INC., publishing as Benjamin Cummings). Reprinted with permission from Ref. [2].*

The superficial epidermis layer of the skin is composed of several types of cells such as keratinocytes, melanocytes, Langerhan's cells, and Merkel's cells. The most plentiful of these are the keratinocytes, which protect the skin and underlying tissue from external assaults. Melanocytes produce the pigment melanin that protects skin from ultraviolet radiation. Langerhans cells are antigen-presenting cells, derived from the bone marrow and lastly, Merkel's cells function as sensory mechanoreceptors (**Figure 2**) [4]. Within the epidermis, the keratinocytes are organized into five strata that undergo morphological and biochemical differentiation until they are shed from the surface of the skin. The deepest of these strata is the stratum basale, which is a single layer of mitotically active cuboidal cells. They undergo either symmetric cell division to promote lateral expansion that provides the regenerative capability of the epidermis, or asymmetric cell division to enable vertical expansion through the production of differentiated keratinocytes [5, 6]. The stratum basale is attached to the basement membrane that separates the epidermis from the other layers of the skin by junctional complexes called hemidesmosomes. Basal keratinocytes move up into the stratum spinosum as they differentiate into the 3–5 layers of the stratum granulosum, where the nuclei flatten. The stratum granulosum keratinocytes contain granules that release lipids contained within lamellar bodies to repel water. Superficial to the stratum granulosum, the stratum lucidum is composed of 3–5 layers of terminally differentiating and flattened keratinocytes. Finally, the outer most layers of the stratum corneum are made up of flat anucleate squames filled with highly cross-linked proteins that help to reduce water loss from skin. These squames slough from the surface and are continuously regenerated (**Figure 2**) [7].

Cells originating at the stratum basale differentiate as they move to more superficial layers and eventually slough off. Thus, the normal function of the skin for protection from chemical, biological, or physiological insults requires a closely coordinated

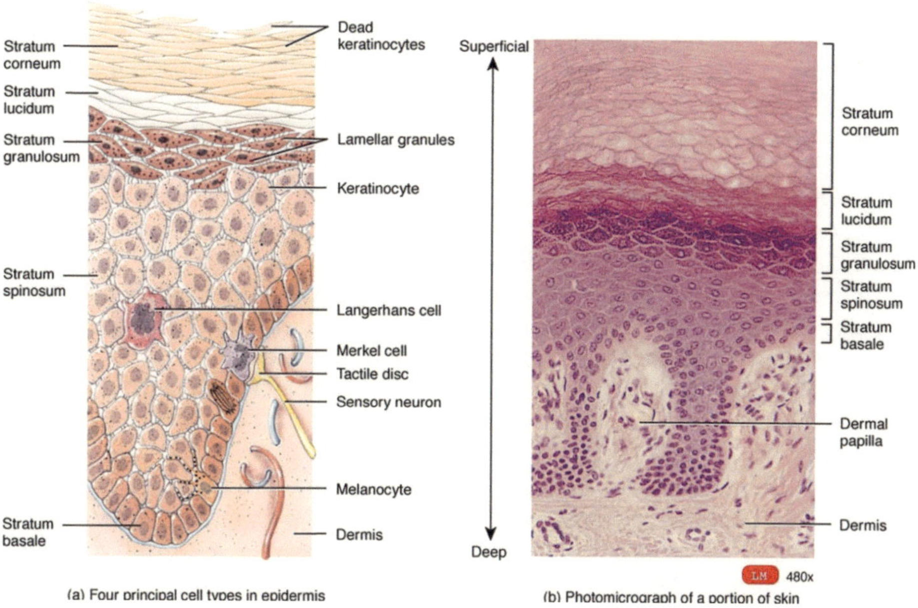


**Figure 2.**
*The structural features of the epidermis (Copyright @ 2007 Pearson Education, INC., publishing as Benjamin Cummings). Reprinted with permission from Ref. [2].*

regulation of proliferation and differentiation. Disruption of this process, through the deregulation of cell cycle pathways, can lead to cancer and other pathologies [8].

### 1.2 Skin cancer

Skin cancer is common among those with outdoor jobs and has been associated with excessive sun exposure ever since the nineteenth century. The incidence of skin cancer is high in populations with light skin and its occurrence has increased over the years, where more than 1.2 million skin cancers occur worldwide each year [9]. Skin cancer is classified into two main types: melanoma and non-melanoma skin cancer. Each year, the incidence of non-melanomas surpasses the combined incidence of cancers of the breast, prostate, lung, and colon together [10]. Non-melanoma skin cancers are not reported to cancer registries due to their early detection and low mortality rates. They rarely metastasize beyond the original tumor site and are seldom fatal but can be extremely detrimental if untreated [10]. The most common type among these is basal cell carcinoma (BCC) followed by squamous cell carcinoma (SCC) [11]. The latter type results from the abnormal growth of the epithelial cells of the epidermis and is more aggressive than BCCs because of their potential to invade and metastasize if kept untreated. Squamous cell carcinoma of the skin metastasizes about 5% of the time in primary tumors of sun-exposed skin with a higher rate for primary SCCs in non-exposed areas of skin [12, 13]. SCC accounts for less than 0.1% of all cancer deaths [14, 15] and is 65 to 250 times more common in immunosuppressed transplant patients, in which it presents with much more aggressive characteristics, more frequent recurrence, and higher likelihood of metastasis [16].

Merkel cell carcinoma is a rare type of non-melanoma skin cancer with a steady incidence rate, yet highly aggressive and fast growing [17]. It is also known as neuroendocrine carcinoma of the skin due to the fact that Merkel cells are connected to the nerve endings and responsible for sensory. Other rare types of non-melanomas include T-cell lymphoma and Kaposi's sarcoma found in older individuals [18].

Melanoma skin cancer, on the other hand, is less common but more deadly since it can grow more deeply below within the skin layers and travel through the lymphatic system and metastasize. In the past decade, the number of melanoma skin cancer cases increased by 27%. Once melanoma spreads deeper into the skin and invades to other parts of the body, it becomes difficult to treat and has less survival rates [19]. Early experiments indicated the effect of UV radiation on DNA damage leading to mutations [20] and that skin pigmentation had a protective effect against skin cancer. The main etiological trigger of skin cancers is contributed to cumulative exposure to UV radiation [21].

Other risk factors include older age, Human papillomavirus infection, exposure to chemicals like arsenic, which is found naturally in water in some areas, genetic predisposition, immunosuppression, and having a fair complexion. Melanin is the protective pigment in the outer epidermis layer, which helps protect the skin from ultraviolet (UV) radiation. Therefore, fair-skinned people, who produce less melanin, are particularly susceptible to developing skin cancer [15]. Similarly, to other cancers, skin cancer is caused by a genetic alteration that leads to uncontrolled division and growth of cells.

## 2. Ultraviolet radiation is a main carcinogen for skin cancer

Ultraviolet radiation (UVR) spectrum of the sunlight is the major cause in the development of skin cancers. UVR is subdivided into: Ultraviolet A (UVA) with a wavelength range of (315-400 nm), Ultraviolet B (280–315 nm), and ultraviolet C (100–280 nm). Among these types, 95% UVA and 5% UVB radiation reach the earth and can penetrate the skin due to their infiltration by the ozone layer of the atmosphere [22]. UVB radiation tempts to burn the skin at a much lower dose than UVA and creates a higher risk for skin cancer. Due to the exhaustion of the ozone levels by environmental pollutions, the atmosphere continues to lose more of its protective filter function; hence, more UVB radiation reaches the earth's surface, increasing the risk of UVR penetrating the skin [23].

The depth of UV radiation penetrating the skin is correlated with its wavelength. UVA, with the longest wavelength, penetrates furthest into the skin, causing damage to both the epidermis and dermis. UVB has a shorter wavelength and typically does not reach past the epidermis layer; however, it is more effective in causing sunburns and skin cancer. UVC rays are normally filtered by the atmospheric ozone layer and therefore do not usually contribute to skin cancer.

Additionally, indoor tanning devices can emit UV radiation 10-15 times higher than direct sun exposure and exert their effect through the emission of both UVA and UVB radiation. Several studies have associated indoor tanning with an increased risk of melanoma and non-melanoma skin cancers [24, 25]. People with less protective melanin pigmentation have a high tendency to accumulate skin burns, which can stimulate skin cancer development.

## 3. Pathogenesis of skin cancer

UV radiation was known to induce skin cancer since the nineteenth century, but it was not until the 1940s when it became evident that UV induced DNA damage. Later in the 1970s, oncogenes and tumor suppressor genes were further discovered to be related to skin cancer development [26]. The carcinogenicity of UVA and UVB radiation includes the process of direct photochemical damage of DNA in the form of cyclobutene pyrimidine dimers (CPDs) and 6–4 photoproducts (6–4 PPs). UVB and UVA also cause oxidative stress associated with increased production of oxidizing species such as 8-oxo-7,8-dihydroguanine (8-oxoG), which can also lead to mutations [27]. It also includes activation of the inflammatory processes and suppression of cutaneous antitumor immunity [28].

UV-induced DNA damage leads to a cell cycle arrest at the G1/S and G2/M checkpoints. This allows the cell to repair any damage or trigger apoptosis before replication [29]. A major mechanism for the repair of DNA damage is the Nucleotide Excision Repair (NER) and Base Excision Repair (BES) for oxidative damage. These enzymatic pathways recognize and correct UV-induced DNA lesions by cutting out the oligo-containing damage and filling its place with a complementary strand to maintain integrity of the genome. A defect in this mechanism increases the risk of skin cancer. Xeroderma pigmentosum (XP) is a rare autosomal recessive disease in which the NER mechanism is defected and therefore has a 1000-fold increased risk of developing skin cancer (**Figure 3**) [30].

As the UV-induced DNA damage accumulates, mutations occur. Mutations in certain genes contribute to genetic instability and the development and progression of

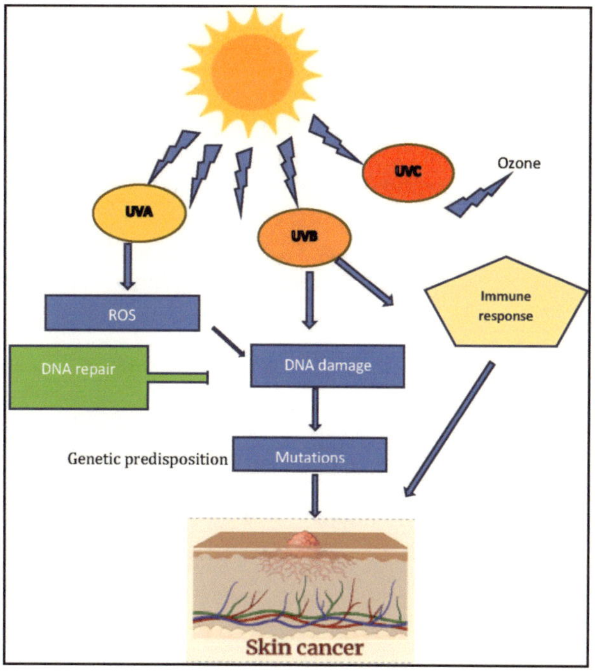


**Figure 3.**
*Pathogenesis of skin cancer (figure created by the author).*

both melanoma and non-melanoma skin cancers in response to the DNA insult [31]. The mutations can activate oncogenes, inactivate tumor suppressor genes, or impair DNA repair genes, all leading to increased proliferation, blood vessel growth, tumor invasion, evasion of immune response, and ultimately, metastasis [31].

### 3.1 Non-melanoma skin cancer pathogenesis

Non-melanoma skin cancers arise *via* a multistep process, gradually acquiring mutations and progressing to precancerous lesions such as actinic keratosis (AK), keratosis, dermatitis, scars, chronic ulcers, or Bowen's disease (BD) [32]. In AK, atypical keratinocytes are present primarily in the basal and less differentiated layers of the epidermis [33]. Bowen's disease and squamous cell carcinoma *in situ* are characterized by atypical keratinocytes throughout the epidermis. These lesions have a 3–5% chance to invade beyond the basement membrane and thus develop into SCC (**Figure 4**) [18, 35].

Recent studies have shown that UVR-induced signal transduction plays a huge role in the initiation and progression of non-melanoma cancer and is remarkably complex. Many signaling pathways are activated and can provoke a suppressive apoptotic response, or an oncogenic pro-survival response according to the duration of exposure to UV and the level of DNA damage. Among the foremost of these signaling pathways are the Ataxia Telangiectasia Mutated (ATM) and RAD3-related (ATR) pathways, where ATM and ATR proteins are recruited by DNA damage sensing proteins [36]. Once recruited at the site of a double-strand break, ATM activates downstream signaling pathways by phosphorylating the effector checkpoint kinases (Chk1 and Chk2) as well as p53. P53, in turn, activates p21 and blocks cyclin-dependent kinase (CDK)/ cyclin E complex activation, leading to cell cycle arrest [37]. Chk1/2 phosphorylate cell division cycle 25 (CDC25) phosphatases, resulting in their degradation.

Progression of non-melanoma skin cancer has been associated with increased activity of Dual specificity cell division cycle 25 (CDC25) phosphatases, which are regulators of cell cycle and apoptosis [38, 39]. It has been shown that ErbB2 is upstream of a DNA damage cell cycle checkpoint and is activated following UV irradiation [40, 41]. This activation signals the PI3K/Akt pathway, which results in the inhibitory phosphorylation of Chk1 on $Ser^{280}$. This blocks the activation of Chk2, thereby inhibiting the phosphorylation of CDC25A and leading to its sustained function, which can increase tumor progression [42]. Increased expression of CDC25

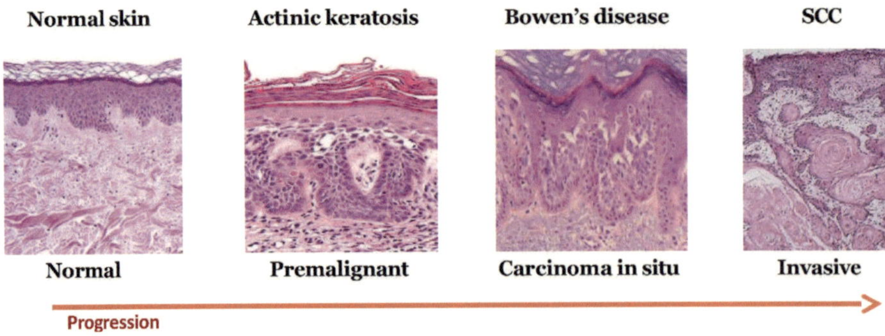


**Figure 4.**
*SCC development is a multistep process that can involve premalignant actinic keratosis or Bowen's disease. Authors own photos from Ref. [34].*

phosphatases in skin cancer has an anti-apoptotic and pro-survival effect, allowing tumor progression [38]. ATR is recruited at the site of a single-strand break and can also phosphorylate ATM. UVR-induced activation of ATR leads to the phosphorylation of Chk1 on $Ser^{345}$, which subsequently phosphorylates and inhibits the activity of CDC25, resulting in cell cycle arrest in a similar manner to Chk2 [36]. In the presence of reactive oxygen species (ROS), apoptosis signal-regulating kinase1 (*ASK1*) is activated and promotes apoptosis by activating p53 [36]. A cell proliferative response occurs through the activation of PI3K/mTOR and Raf-MEK-ERK pathways downstream of UVR-induced receptor tyrosine kinases.

Common mutations found in cSCC include those in *RAS* oncogene, which encodes RAS protein. This gene plays a crucial role in the evolution of non-melanoma carcinomas through regulation of proliferation, apoptosis, and angiogenesis. Additionally, inactivation of E-cadherin membrane protein, which is involved in epithelial cell adhesion, is associated with the invasion and metastasis of SCC [18]. The SCC is capable of locally infiltrative growth, spreading to regional lymph nodes and leading to distant metastasis, most often to the lungs. Invasive SCC occurs in the epidermis and invades the dermis [43].

BCC, the most common form of non-melanoma cancers, is not aggressive and rarely metastasizes. BCC originates from pluripotent interfollicular stem cells and involves mainly a mutation in the sonic Hedgehog signaling pathway as a result of high exposure to UV radiation in 90% of the cases [44]. *PTCH1* gene, which codes for the sonic hedgehog (SSH) receptor, is mutated and tumorigenesis is induced by opposing cell cycle arrest and differentiation, resulting in uncontrolled cell growth and formation of hyperplasia. Another common affected pathway in BCC is found on the Canonical (β-catenin dependent) Wingless (WNT) signaling pathway [44]. Other common mutations induced by UVR exposure found in BCC are seen in the *P53* tumor suppressive gene [45, 46].

T-cell lymphoma is related to immunosuppression, where there is a marked decrease in T cell lymphocytes, which in turn is caused by the loss of an important receptor, CD28 protein preventing clonal expansion of T cells [47]. Both Merkel's carcinoma and Kaposi's sarcoma are also associated with immune suppression [18].

### 3.2 Melanoma skin cancer pathogenesis

Melanoma originates from pigment-producing melanocytes located in the basal layer of the epidermis. The etiology of melanoma is related to both genetic and environmental factors. The main environmental influence is intermittent intense exposure to UV radiation. Although melanin produced by melanocytes has a protective antioxidant feature against UV-induced damage, this feature can be converted to a pro-oxidant when oxidized by the reactive oxygen species generated from the UV radiation [48]. This in turn leads to the increase of oxidative stress and eventually leads to the acquisition of mutations that can alter the control of the cells and progress to melanoma cancer [49]. The progression of malignant melanoma involves a complex series of pathways and oncogenic targets that interact together. The most frequent of these oncogenic targets is the *v*-Raf murine sarcoma viral oncogene (*BRAF*), which acts in the mitogen-activated protein kinase and extracellular signal-regulated kinase (*MAP/ERK*) pathway involved in the regulation of cell proliferation, cell growth, and migration. Mutations on *BRAF* are found in dysplastic nevi (a clonal population of melanocytes) and lead to nevus development reaching a senescent stage [50].

Further mutations in tumor suppressor genes such as *PTEN and NRAS* will contribute to melanocytes evading senescence, leading to the transformation of the nevus to melanoma confined to the epidermis where radial growth phase occurs (RGP) at early stages. Additionally, inactivation of the tumor suppressors *CDKN2A and P53* aids in the progression and invasion of melanoma, causing the vertical growth phase (VGP) and ultimately metastasis [51, 52].

The PI3K-AKT pathway is another separate signaling pathway that plays a role in melanoma cell proliferation and survival. Phosphatidylinositol-3-kinase (PI3K) is involved in various functions within the cell, such as cell growth and proliferation. It leads to the phosphorylation and activation of the serine-threonine-specific kinase, AKT and elicits progression and a strong anti-apoptotic effect [50].

Melanocytes are normally connected to basal keratinocytes through the transmembrane glycoprotein E-cadherin. When melanoma transitions to the metastatic stage, it undergoes epithelial to mesenchymal transition (EMT), which involves switching the E-cadherin to N-cadherin to be up regulated through the WNT signaling pathway. Subsequently, the newly increased N-cadherin facilitates melanoma migration into the dermis and its interaction with dermal fibroblasts and vascular endothelial cells allowing the spread of melanoma cancer [19].

## 4. Diagnosis of non-melanoma and melanoma skin cancers

Cutaneous SCC can be presented in its early stages as its precursor, actinic keratosis, and can develop to become hyperkeratotic as it progresses. cSCC can also appear as an asymptomatic small plaque or nodule that enlarges over time. It can show in different forms such as crateriform, ulcerated, necrotic, or botryomycotic [53]. BCC is presented as a shiny pink nodule that may enlarge to have an ulcer appearance, most commonly on the nose, cheeks, eyelids, or forehead [54]. Dermoscopy is used to differentiate diagnosis through a biopsy of the lesion. Histologic staining and immunohistochemical markers, such as cytokeratins, are used to confirm diagnosis. The histopathological picture of cSCC shows strands of atypical keratinocytes originating in the epidermis and infiltrating into the dermis [53]. The histopathological picture also displays islands or nests of basaloid cells with basophilic nuclei and scanty cytoplasm [55].

Early detection of melanoma according to clinical features is based on the ABCDE rule, which stands for *A*symmetry of the cancerous lesion, *B*order-irregularity, *C*olor variation of the lesion, *D*iameter of more than 6 mm, and *E*volution of the lesion where it becomes larger or changes in color [56]. Additional confirmation of melanoma diagnosis is through the histological features where melanoma will be classified based on Clark's level (how deep the tumor invades in the skin) and Breslow depth (depth in millimeters of invasion). Accordingly, the four types of melanomas are superficial spreading melanoma (SSM), lentigo maligna melanoma (LMM), nodular melanoma (NM), and acral lentiginous melanoma (ALM) [57]. Furthermore, the tumor is staged to provide information that can guide treatment and prognosis. Imaging tests such as a positron emission tomography (PET) scan and Computed tomography (CT) scan aid in staging the tumor. Stage 0 is given if the tumor is confined to the epidermis and can be treated with surgical excision. Stage 1 is considered early melanoma where the tumor is less than 1 mm in depth. Stage 2 is given if the tumor is between 1 and 4 mm in depth. Stage 3 is when the tumor has spread to nearby lymph nodes. Finally, stage 4 is the most advanced stage, owing to the spread of the tumor to other parts of the body. High blood level of lactate dehydrogenase (LDH) is also found at this stage [58].

Furthermore, recent studies have utilized artificial intelligence using deep learning-driven models to identify and classify skin cancers using dermoscopic images, aiming to improve the accuracy and efficiency of the diagnosis of skin cancers [59, 60].

## 5. Treatment of skin cancer

Treatment options depend on various factors such as size, location of the tumor, possible side effects, and patients' preference.

Surgical excision is the first-line treatment for tumors at the early stages. Non-melanoma and early stages of melanoma mainly rely on surgical removal as a standard of care. Affected regional lymph nodes are dissected to decrease the risk of recurrence. A technique called MOHs micrographic surgery is used when the cancer is a recurrent type. This procedure requires the removal of the tumorous tissue followed by a microscopic analysis during the surgery to histologically assess the area *via* a thin frozen section for any further tumor cells, if so, an additional layer is excised. This is repeated until there are no signs of tumor cells [31].

Cryosurgery and Radiation therapy may be used for areas that are difficult to perform surgery on, such as the non-melanoma cancer on the eyelid. It can also be given as an additional preventive treatment after surgery [61]. Another treatment used for lesions located on the surface of the skin is Photodynamic therapy (PDT), which transforms light energy into heat energy. The area is exposed to a special wavelength of light after applying a topical medication containing aminolevulinic acid, producing cytotoxic effects that leads to the damage of the function of targeted tumor cells and subsequently their death. Studies have shown that PDT is effective for BCC and can help prevent the development of SCC [31].

Immune therapy is a novel approach widely used to treat skin cancers, mainly melanoma since it is an immunogenic tumor. Interferons, a group of signaling cytokines that induce protection against disorders, play an important role in immunotherapy against cancer. They induce an antitumor response by producing anti-proliferative effects [62]. Types of immune therapy include Cytokine therapy and cancer vaccines, which enhance the immune response against cancer cells. Checkpoint inhibitors such as Programmed cell death protein 1 (PD-1) and cytotoxic T-Lymphocyte-associated protein 4(CTLA-4) are other types of immune therapy. These inhibitors block the inhibition of immune response allowing immune cells to detect and attack cancer cells [31]. An alternative more personalized immune therapy approach is the Chimeric Antigen Receptor T-cell therapy (CAR-T), which involves genetically modifying the patients' T-Cells to express receptors to target skin cancer [63]. Topical immune therapy can be used, such as ingenol mebutate (IM), which promotes anti-tumor antibodies [64].

Chemotherapy can be topically applied on tumors where several lesions are spread across various sites on the body or when they are poor candidates of surgical removal. Topical 5-fluorouracil (5-FU) chemotherapy is commonly used for BCC. Other topical treatments include retinoid, which was also shown to have a chemo-preventive effect on BCC. A more recent treatment, being explored for patients with advanced BCC, is the Hedgehog pathway inhibitors [65].

An emerging approach in the treatment of metastasized skin cancer is through nanotechnology that operates at a nanoscale and can help in tumor imaging and can increase drug delivery and distribution in the body. Quantum dots are nanocrystals with optical and electric properties and may be functionalized with antibodies that target skin cancer cells. With the emission of light from these dots, it would help the clinicians in precisely identifying the areas of cancer cells. Nanoparticles can also be applied to deliver drug to specific cancer cells. The first-line treatment for advanced melanoma is dacarbazine (DTIC), which can be delivered via nanoparticles [66]. Due to its heterogeneity and variation in mutations and affected pathways, skin cancer has potential to develop and worsen. Therefore, single choice of treatments may be challenging, and the need of combination therapy is required. This involves pairing therapies such as immunotherapy with radiation therapy, to hence decrease recurrence and increase survival [67].

## 6. Conclusion

Rapid globalization has led to continuous depletion of the ozone layer allowing more entry of UVA and UVB to the earth, which in turn leads to more genetic alterations in the skin cells, leading to increased incidents of skin cancer. Although skin cancer mortality rates are low, the high incidence in countries of Caucasians results in a high-cost burden. DNA repair response to UV-induced damage in the skin is very important. The molecular signaling mechanisms during skin carcinogenesis are extremely complex and depend on the intensity and duration of UV-induced damage. This mechanism can induce either oncogenic or tumor suppression effects with extensive crosstalk between pathways. Furthermore, genetic variation between individuals can further introduce the complexity of signaling pathways and hence treatment response. Prevention and early diagnosis are must through increasing awareness of the harmful effects of sun exposure and indoor tanning beds, and the importance of utilization of sun protection. This concludes the significance of early screening protocols for high-risk populations through a complete skin examination.

## Abbreviations

| | |
|---|---|
| UVR | ultraviolet radiation |
| BCC | basal cell carcinoma |
| SCC | squamous cell carcinoma |
| CPDs | cyclobutene pyrimidine dimers |
| 6–4 PPs | 6–4 photoproducts |
| 8-oxoG | 8-oxo- 7,8-dihydroguanine |
| AK | actinic keratosis |
| BD | Bowen's disease |
| ATM | Ataxia telangiectasia |
| ATR | RAD3-related |
| Chk1 and Chk2 | checkpoint kinases |
| CDK | cyclin-dependent kinase |
| CDC25 | cell division cycle 25 |
| *BRAF* | *v*-Raf murine sarcoma viral oncogene |
| *MAP/ERK* | mitogen-activated protein kinase and extracellular signal-regulated kinase |
| ROS | reactive oxygen species |
| *ASK1* | apoptosis signal-regulating kinase1 |
| PI3K/mTOR | phosphoinositide 3-kinase/mechanistic target of rapamycin |

*DOI: http://dx.doi.org/10.5772/intechopen.1005790*

| | |
|---|---|
| SSH | Sonic Hedgehog |
| *PTCH1* | protein patched homolog 1 |
| WNT | canonical (β-catenin dependent) wingless |
| *PTEN* | phosphatase and tensin homolog |
| VGP | vertical growth phase |
| RGP | radial growth phase |
| EMT | epithelial to mesenchymal transition |
| SSM | superficial spreading melanoma |
| LMM | lentigo maligna melanoma |
| NM | nodular melanoma |
| ALM | acral lentiginous |
| PD-1 | programmed cell death protein |
| CTLA-4 | cytotoxic T-lymphocyte-associated protein 4 |
| CAR-T | chimeric antigen receptor T-cell therapy |

## Author details

Jenan Al-Matouq
Mohammed Al-Mana College for Medical Science, Dammam, Saudi Arabia

*Address all correspondence to: jenana@machs.edu.sa

## References


[1] Forslind B, Lindberg M. Skin, Hair, and Nails: Structure and Function. Informa Healthcare; 2003

[2] Marieb EN, Hoehn K. In: Marieb EN, Hoehn K, editors. Human Anatomy and Physiology. 2016

[3] Kanitakis J. Anatomy, histology and immunohistochemistry of normal human skin. European Journal of Dermatology. 2002;**12**(4):390-399; quiz 400-1

[4] Bouwstra JA, Pilgram GSK, Ponec M. Skin Barrier. In: Elias PM, Feingold KR, editors. 1st ed. Boca Raton: CRC Press; 2005

[5] Montagna W. Cutaneous comparative biology. Archives of Dermatology. 1971;**104**:6

[6] Lavker RM, Sun TT. Heterogeneity in epidermal basal keratinocytes: Morphological and functional correlations. Science. 1979, 1982;**215**(4537):1239-1241

[7] O'Rahilly R, Montagna W. The structure and function of skin. The Quarterly Review of Biology. 1974;(3):18-74

[8] Noell C, Aleissa S, Nguyen BM. Skin Cancer: At-Risk Populations and Prevention. In: A Practical Guide to Skin Cancer. Cham: Springer International Publishing; 2018. pp. 1-20

[9] Ferlay J, Colombet M, Soerjomataram I, Parkin DM, Piñeros M, Znaor A, et al. Cancer statistics for the year 2020: An overview. International Journal of Cancer. 2021;**149**(4):778-789

[10] Kivisaari A, Kähäri VM. Squamous cell carcinoma of the skin: Emerging need for novel biomarkers. World Journal of Clinical Oncology. 2013;**4**(4):85-90

[11] Rogers HW, Weinstock MA, Feldman SR, Coldiron BM. Incidence estimate of nonmelanoma skin cancer (keratinocyte carcinomas) in the U.S. population, 2012. JAMA Dermatology. 2015;**151**(10):1081-1086

[12] Ao R, Fu R, Dong D, Zhu X, Liu H, Xie K. Discerning primary tumors from metastases in synchronous nasopharyngeal squamous cell carcinoma and cutaneous squamous cell carcinoma: A case report and review of the literature. Oncology Letters. 2014;**7**(5):1391-1394

[13] Fitzpatrick TB, Wolff K, Goldsmith LA, Katz SI, Gilchrest BA, Paller AS, et al. Fitzpatrick's Dermatology in General Medicine. 7th ed. New York: McGraw Hill Medical Access Medicine Clinical Library; 2008

[14] Gordon R. Skin cancer: An overview of epidemiology and risk factors. Seminars in Oncology Nursing. 2013;**29**(3):160-169

[15] Euvrard S, Kanitakis J, Claudy A. Skin cancers after organ transplantation. The New England Journal of Medicine. 2003;**348**(17):1681-1691

[16] Armstrong BK, Kricker A. The epidemiology of UV induced skin cancer. Journal of Photochemistry and Photobiology. B. 2001;**63**(1-3):8-18

[17] Brady M, Spiker AM. Cancer, Merkel cell of the skin. In: StatPearls. Treasure Island (Fl): StatPearls Publishing; 2019

[18] Souto EB, da Ana R, Vieira V, Fangueiro JF, Dias-Ferreira J, Cano A, et al. Non-melanoma skin cancers: Physio-

pathology and role of lipid delivery systems in new chemotherapeutic treatments. Neoplasia. 2022;**30**:100810

[19] Liu Y, Sheikh MS. Melanoma: Molecular pathogenesis and therapeutic management. Molecular and Cellular Pharmacology. 2014;**6**(3):228

[20] Hollaender A, Emmons CW. Wavelength dependence of mutation production in the ultraviolet with special emphasis on fungi. In: Cold Spring Harbor Symposia on Quantitative Biology. 1 Jan 1941;**9**(0):179-186

[21] Boukamp P. Non-melanoma skin cancer: What drives tumor development and progression? Carcinogenesis. 2005;**26**(10):1657-1667

[22] Narayanan DL, Saladi RN, Fox JL. Ultraviolet radiation and skin cancer. International Journal of Dermatology. 2010;**49**(9):978-986

[23] El Ghissassi F, Baan R, Straif K, Grosse Y, Secretan B, Bouvard V, et al. A review of human carcinogens–Part D: Radiation. The Lancet Oncology. 2009;**10**(8):751-752

[24] Le Clair MZ, Cockburn MG. Tanning bed use and melanoma: Establishing risk and improving prevention interventions. Preventive Medical Reports. 2016;**3**:139-144

[25] Bataille V, Winnett A, Sasieni P, Newton Bishop JA, Cuzick J. Exposure to the sun and sunbeds and the risk of cutaneous melanoma in the UK: A case-control study. European Journal of Cancer. 2004;**40**(3):429-35

[26] Falto-Aizpurua L, Griffth R, Simmons B, Nouri K. The history of skin cancer. Journal of the American Academy of Dermatology. 2015;**72**(5):AB27

[27] Rass K, Reichrath J. UV damage and DNA repair in malignant melanoma and nonmelanoma skin cancer. Advances in Experimental Medicine and Biology. 2008;**624**:162-178

[28] Snaidr VA, Damian DL, Halliday GM. Nicotinamide for photoprotection and skin cancer chemoprevention: A review of efficacy and safety. Experimental Dermatology. 2019;**28**(Suppl. 1):15-22

[29] Tomescu D, Kavanagh G, Ha T, Campbell H, Melton DW. Nucleotide excision repair gene XPD polymorphisms and genetic predisposition to melanoma. Carcinogenesis. 2001;**22**(3):403-408

[30] Emmert S, Kraemer KH. Do not underestimate nucleotide excision repair: It predicts not only melanoma risk but also survival outcome. The Journal of Investigative Dermatology. 2013;**133**(7):1713-1717

[31] Hasan N, Nadaf A, Imran M, Jiba U, Sheikh A, Almalki WH, et al. Skin cancer: Understanding the journey of transformation from conventional to advanced treatment approaches. Molecular Cancer. 2023;**22**(1):168

[32] Anand R, Mallipeddi R. Mohs Surgery. In: Non-melanoma Skin Cancer: Essentials for Oncologists. Boca Raton: CRC Press; 2023

[33] Neubert T, Lehmann P. Bowen's disease - A review of newer treatment options. Therapeutics and Clinical Risk Management. 2008;**4**(5):1085-1095

[34] Almatouq J. Role of CDC25 phosphatases in non-melanoma skin cancer [doctoral]. Omaha: Creighton University; 2014

[35] Yanofsky VR, Mercer SE, Phelps RG. Histopathological variants of cutaneous

squamous cell carcinoma: A review. Journal of Skin Cancer. 2011;**2011**:1-13

[36] Feehan RP, Shantz LM. Molecular signaling cascades involved in nonmelanoma skin carcinogenesis. The Biochemical Journal. 2016;**473**(19):2973-2994

[37] Stokes MP, Rush J, Macneill J, Ren JM, Sprott K, Nardone J, et al. Profiling of UV-induced ATM/ATR signaling pathways. Proceedings of the National Academy of Sciences of the United States of America. 2007;**104**(50):19855-19860

[38] Al-Matouq J, Holmes T, Hammiller B, Tran N, Holmes M, Freeman SC, et al. Accumulation of cytoplasmic CDC25A in cutaneous squamous cell carcinoma leads to a dependency on CDC25A for cancer cell survival and tumor growth. Cancer Letters. 2017;**410**:41-49

[39] Al-Matouq J, Holmes TR, Hansen LA. CDC25B and CDC25C overexpression in nonmelanoma skin cancer suppresses cell death. Molecular Carcinogenesis. 2019;**58**(9):1691-1700

[40] Reddy JP, Peddibhotla S, Bu W, Zhao J, Haricharan S, Du YCN, et al. Defining the ATM-mediated barrier to tumorigenesis in somatic mammary cells following ErbB2 activation. Proceedings of the National Academy of Sciences of the United States of America. 2010;**107**(8):3728-3733

[41] Madson JG, Lynch DT, Svoboda J, Ophardt R, Yanagida J, Putta SK, et al. Erbb2 suppresses DNA damage-induced checkpoint activation and UV-induced mouse skin tumorigenesis. The American Journal of Pathology. 2009;**174**(6):2357-2366

[42] Kvam E, Tyrrell RM. Induction of oxidative DNA base damage in human skin cells by UV and near visible radiation. Carcinogenesis. 1997;**18**(12):2379-2384

[43] Josiah AJ, Twilley D, Pillai SK, Ray SS, Lall N. Pathogenesis of keratinocyte carcinomas and the therapeutic potential of medicinal plants and phytochemicals. Molecules. 2021;**26**(7):1979

[44] Kashyap MP, Sinha R, Mukhtar MS, Athar M. Epigenetic regulation in the pathogenesis of non-melanoma skin cancer. Seminars in Cancer Biology. 2022;**83**:36-56

[45] Lesiak A, Sobolewska-Sztychny D, Majak P, Sobjanek M, Wodz K, Sygut KP, et al. Relation between sonic hedgehog pathway gene polymorphisms and basal cell carcinoma development in the polish population. Archives of Dermatological Research. 2016;**308**(1):39-47

[46] Kilgour JM, Jia JL, Sarin KY. Review of the molecular genetics of basal cell carcinoma; inherited susceptibility, somatic mutations, and targeted therapeutics. Cancers (Basel). 2021;**13**(15):3870

[47] Schrom KP, Kim I, Baron ED. The immune system and pathogenesis of melanoma and non-melanoma skin cancer. Advances in Experimental Medicine and Biology. 2020;**1268**:211-226

[48] Meyskens FL Jr, Farmer PJ, Anton-Culver H. Etiologic pathogenesis of melanoma: A unifying hypothesis for the missing attributable risk. Clinical Cancer Research. 2004;**10**(8):2581-2583

[49] Strashilov S, Yordanov A. Aetiology and pathogenesis of cutaneous melanoma: Current concepts and advances. International Journal of Molecular Sciences. 2021;**22**(12):6395

[50] Paluncic J, Kovacevic Z, Jansson PJ, Kalinowski D, Merlot AM, Huang MLH,

et al. Roads to melanoma: Key pathways and emerging players in melanoma progression and oncogenic signaling. Biochimica et Biophysica Acta. 2016;**1863**(4):770-784

[51] Shreberk-Hassidim R, Ostrowski SM, Fisher DE. The complex interplay between Nevi and melanoma: Risk factors and precursors. International Journal of Molecular Sciences. 2023;**24**(4):3541

[52] Zaidi MR, Day CP, Merlino G. From UVs to metastases: Modeling melanoma initiation and progression in the mouse. The Journal of Investigative Dermatology. 2008;**128**(10):2381-2391

[53] Stratigos A, Garbe C, Lebbe C, Malvehy J, del Marmol V, Pehamberger H, et al. Diagnosis and treatment of invasive squamous cell carcinoma of the skin: European consensus-based interdisciplinary guideline. European Journal of Cancer. 2015;**51**(14):1989-2007

[54] Marzuka AG, Book SE. Basal cell carcinoma: Pathogenesis, epidemiology, clinical features, diagnosis, histopathology, and management. Yale Journal of Biology and Medicine. 2015;**88**(2):167-179

[55] Mackiewicz-Wysocka M, Bowszyc-Dmochowska M, Strzelecka-Węklar D, Dańczak-Pazdrowska A, Adamski Z. Reviews basal cell carcinoma – Diagnosis. Współczesna Onkologia. 2013;**4**:337-342

[56] Abbasi NR, Shaw HM, Rigel DS, Friedman RJ, McCarthy WH, Osman I, et al. Early diagnosis of cutaneous melanoma: Revisiting the ABCD criteria. Journal of the American Medical Association. 2004 Dec;**292**(22):2771-2776

[57] Davis LE, Shalin SC, Tackett AJ. Current state of melanoma diagnosis and treatment. Cancer Biology & Therapy. 2019;**20**(11):1366-1379

[58] Swetter SM, Tsao H, Bichakjian CK, Curiel-Lewandrowski C, Elder DE, Gershenwald JE, et al. Guidelines of care for the management of primary cutaneous melanoma. Journal of the American Academy of Dermatology. 2019;**80**(1):208-250

[59] Malibari AA, Alzahrani JS, Eltahir MM, Malik V, Obayya M, Al DM, et al. Optimal deep neural network-driven computer aided diagnosis model for skin cancer. Computers and Electrical Engineering. 2022;**103**:108318

[60] Zhang L, Zhang J, Gao W, Bai F, Li N, Ghadimi N. A deep learning outline aimed at prompt skin cancer detection utilizing gated recurrent unit networks and improved orca predation algorithm. Biomedical Signal Processing and Control. 2024;**90**:105858

[61] Choudhary S, Tang J, Elsaie ML, Nouri K. Lasers in the treatment of nonmelanoma skin cancer. Dermatologic Surgery. 2011;**37**(4):409-425

[62] Amini S, Viera MH, Valins W, Berman B. Nonsurgical innovations in the treatment of nonmelanoma skin cancer. Journal of Clinical and Aesthetic Dermatology. 2010;**3**(6):20-34

[63] Mellman I, Coukos G, Dranoff G. Cancer immunotherapy comes of age. Nature. 2011;**480**(7378):480-489

[64] Voiculescu VM, Lisievici CV, Lupu M, Vajaitu C, Draghici CC, Popa AV, et al. Mediators of inflammation in topical therapy of skin cancers. Mediators of Inflammation. 2019;**2019**:8369690

[65] Gambini D, Passoni E, Nazzaro G, Beltramini G, Tomasello G, Ghidini M,

et al. Basal cell carcinoma and Hedgehog pathway inhibitors: Focus on immune response. Frontiers in Medicine (Lausanne). 2022;**9**:893063

[66] Dianzani C, Zara GP, Maina G, Pettazzoni P, Pizzimenti S, Rossi F, et al. Drug delivery nanoparticles in skin cancers. BioMed Research International. 2014;**2014**:895986

[67] Bhatia K, Bhumika DA. Combinatorial drug therapy in cancer - New insights. Life Sciences. 2020;**258**:118134

Chapter 2

# Epidemiology of Skin Cancer in 2024

*Serena Federico, Francesco Fortarezza, Giuseppe Ingravallo and Gerardo Cazzato*

## Abstract

The incidence of skin cancer has risen globally in recent years, with 2024 marking a critical point in understanding its epidemiology and burden on public health. As one of the most common malignancies worldwide, skin cancer results from a combination of genetic predisposition, lifestyle behaviors, environmental exposures, and socioeconomic factors. This chapter provides a comprehensive overview of the current epidemiology of skin cancer, focusing on both melanoma and non-melanoma skin cancers (NMSC). It examines variations in incidence and prevalence across different regions and demographic groups, shedding light on key risk factors such as UV exposure, skin type, geographic location, and evolving trends in sun exposure. The chapter highlights the public health importance of early detection and preventative measures, which are essential to reducing morbidity and mortality associated with skin cancer. The chapter also addresses significant trends, including a marked increase in melanoma among younger populations, particularly in high-UV regions, as well as disparities in access to healthcare that impact skin cancer outcomes. In addition to exploring global NMSC epidemiology—with emphasis on basal cell carcinoma (BCC) and squamous cell carcinoma (SCC) patterns across continents—this chapter reviews the high incidence rates of NMSC in countries like Australia and New Zealand and contrasts them with regions where incidence is lower but mortality rates may be disproportionately high due to limited healthcare access. In discussing melanoma, the chapter analyzes the "divergent pathway" model of tumorigenesis, anatomical site-specific trends, and improvements in diagnostic accuracy due to advances in dermoscopy. Emerging therapeutic options, such as immunotherapies for advanced melanoma, are also explored within the context of reducing melanoma mortality. This chapter thus provides healthcare professionals, researchers, and policymakers with an updated framework for understanding the complexities and pressing needs in skin cancer prevention and management in 2024.

**Keywords:** epidemiology, NMSC, melanoma, skin, neoplasms, overview

## 1. Introduction

In 2024, the growing worldwide incidence of skin cancer is a significant public health problem. Skin cancer is one of the most common types of cancer in the world and is caused by intricate relationships between genetics, personal behavior, environmental factors, and socioeconomic status. Our understanding of skin cancer epidemiology is changing as a result of advancements in public health research, as well as a greater awareness of the roles played by UV radiation, climate change, and demographic trends. An updated summary of the incidence, prevalence, and trends of skin malignancies, including melanoma and non-melanoma skin cancers, in different groups is provided in this chapter. It looks at the effects of risk factors such as skin type, geography, and changing sun-exposure habits, emphasizing the value of early detection and prevention measures in reducing the disease's effects.

This chapter will also cover current epidemiological trends, such as the rising prevalence of melanoma in younger people, especially in areas with high UV exposure, and inequalities in healthcare access that impact diagnostic and treatment results. In order to give healthcare professionals, researchers, and public health policymakers a thorough grasp of the current situation and the obstacles facing the reduction of skin cancer morbidity and mortality, this chapter examines the most recent findings and projections in skin cancer epidemiology.

## 2. Epidemiology of non-melanoma skin cancer worldwide: An updated overview

Non-melanoma skin cancer (NMSC) refers to a group of cancers that originate from the skin's epidermal cells, with the two most common types being basal cell carcinoma (BCC) and squamous cell carcinoma (SCC). NMSC is the most frequently diagnosed cancer globally, with an increasing incidence in both developed and developing nations. This rise is largely attributed to aging populations, increased exposure to ultraviolet (UV) radiation, and improved detection practices. Understanding the global epidemiology of NMSC is crucial for public health efforts aimed at prevention and management. Here, we explore the prevalence, risk factors, and trends in various regions of the world, based on the latest scientific evidence [1, 2].

### 2.1 Global incidence and prevalence

#### *2.1.1 North America*

In North America, particularly the United States and Canada, NMSC incidence is notably high. The United States alone accounts for approximately 5.4 million cases of NMSC annually [3]. BCC is the more common subtype, representing around 80% of cases, while SCC accounts for the remaining 20% [4]. NMSC rates have increased significantly over the last several decades, with studies showing that the incidence of BCC has risen by 145% and SCC by 263% between the 1970s and the 2010s [5]. This trend is largely due to increased sun exposure, the aging population, and greater awareness and early detection. Canada has seen similar trends, though the incidence is lower in its northern provinces due to less UV exposure [6].

#### *2.1.2 Europe*

In Europe, NMSC is also one of the most commonly diagnosed cancers, though incidence varies by region. Northern European countries such as Norway, Sweden, and Denmark report lower rates of NMSC compared to southern countries like Italy,

Spain, and Greece, where higher UV radiation exposure is a significant risk factor [7]. The European Academy of Dermatology and Venereology (EADV) has reported an annual increase of 3–8% in NMSC cases over recent decades [8]. Recent data suggest that the overall incidence of NMSC in Europe may exceed 300 cases per 100,000 people annually [9].

### *2.1.3 Australia and New Zealand*

Australia and New Zealand have the highest reported rates of NMSC in the world, with Australia recording an incidence of over 1000 cases per 100,000 people per year [10]. This region's population is predominantly of European descent, with lighter skin types more susceptible to UV-induced skin damage. The high incidence is largely attributed to the country's proximity to the equator, resulting in higher UV exposure, as well as the widespread outdoor lifestyle and historical underuse of sun protection. In New Zealand, similar factors contribute to high NMSC rates, though public health campaigns have somewhat mitigated the rise [11]. Both countries have been at the forefront of skin cancer prevention campaigns, which have had some success in raising awareness and promoting sun protection.

### *2.1.4 Asia*

In Asia, the incidence of NMSC is generally lower than in Western countries, though it is on the rise in some regions. Countries such as Japan, China, and South Korea have reported increasing rates of NMSC, particularly in urban areas with higher exposure to UV radiation due to lifestyle changes [12]. However, darker skin phototypes common in Asian populations tend to offer some protection against UV-induced skin damage, resulting in lower incidence rates compared to regions with predominantly fair-skinned populations. In South Asia, countries like India and Pakistan report a relatively low incidence of NMSC, though SCC is more prevalent due to the combination of UV exposure and other risk factors like chronic arsenic exposure from contaminated water sources [13].

### *2.1.5 Africa*

NMSC incidence in Africa is lower than in regions with predominantly lighter-skinned populations, although the data are limited. In Sub-Saharan Africa, the incidence of NMSC remains low, largely due to the higher levels of melanin in the skin, which provides natural protection against UV damage. However, in Northern Africa, where fair-skinned individuals are more common, the incidence is higher, and sun exposure is a significant risk factor [14]. Additionally, individuals with albinism in Africa have a substantially higher risk of developing SCC, often at a young age, due to their lack of melanin. Public health efforts to protect this vulnerable population from excessive sun exposure remain critical.

## 3. Epidemiology of melanoma

Skin malignancies are the most frequently diagnosed type of cancer worldwide, with an expected 1.5 million new cases since 2020 [15]. Approximately 1 in 5 of these cancers are represented by melanomas, with a predicted 325,000 cases globally in

2020 alone [15]. Over the past 50 years, melanoma incidence rates have been increasing in people of European descent with fair phenotypes. More than three-quarters of all newly diagnosed melanoma cases can be linked to UV radiation, making populations susceptible to this strong and widespread risk factor for the disease largely responsible for this increase [16]. According to this epidemiological study [17], melanoma represented a substantial portion of the cancer burden in 2020 and was primarily found in highly developed nations that were more vulnerable to the harmful effects of sunlight radiation. Incidence and mortality rates varied significantly by country and region, with the highest incidence found in light-skinned populations in North America, western and northern Europe (including Denmark, Norway, and the Netherlands), and Australia/New Zealand. Melanoma, on the other hand, is still uncommon in many regions of Asia, South and Central America, and Africa. Mortality is out of proportion to incidence in Asia and Africa. Even if there aren't many melanoma cases in developing countries, the disease's death rate is frequently disproportionate, as seen in most of Asia and Africa, most likely as a result of increased mortality rates. Due to the absence of sufficient screening programs in developing nations, where low incidence is linked to disproportionately higher mortality than in nations where incidence is significantly higher due to a higher number of diagnoses in a population that has become more sensitive as a result of ongoing screening campaigns, the various estimates of incidence are severely biased. Due to improvements in therapy, the total mortality rate from melanoma in the United States has decreased significantly over the last ten years (2011–2020), by about 5% annually for those under 50 and 3% annually for those 50 and older. It was anticipated that the disease would be the cause of 7990 deaths in 2023 (5420 men and 2570 women). Between 2007 and 2016, the melanoma death rate decreased by about 2 percent annually for people aged 50 and over and by about 4% annually for those under 50. Public education may have an impact on early discovery and treatment, as evidenced by the decrease in mortality observed in younger patients [17].

Regarding the different anatomical sites, the melanomas of the trunk had the largest increase in incidence, while those of the head and neck had the least; the increases were more pronounced in the female sex for those of the legs. Young females are frequently diagnosed with melanoma in the lower limbs. Although it is still better than other localizations, the prognosis is dependent on age, histological subtype, and concurrent genetic and environmental variables. The "divergent pathway" model, which explains the idea that people who are more likely to develop fewer melanocytic nevi need more sun exposure to encourage the development of melanoma, and that they are more likely to develop melanoma on areas of their bodies that are exposed to the sun on a regular basis, like their head or neck, is taken into account today [18]. On the other hand, those who have a lot of nevi may need less sun exposure to promote the growth of melanoma, and they are more likely to have melanoma in areas like the back where there are a lot of nevi. According to this "divergent pathway" paradigm, melanomas may develop on various body parts through distinct pathways [16].

Thanks to the numerous studies that correlate dermoscopic patterns with specific histological characteristics of melanoma, the diagnostic accuracy of clinical diagnosis has greatly increased [19]. The aim of clinical diagnosis is early detection in the *in situ* stage of melanoma and the increase in the global incidence of melanoma in recent years is due to a growing and increasing diagnostic sensitivity [18, 19]. The increase in the prevalence of melanoma as a systemic disease is due to new therapeutic opportunities implemented within the framework of multidisciplinary management of a pathology that today, for genetic and environmental reasons, becomes more frequent.

Taking into account that already in stage IIb-IIc, immunotherapy can be considered, of course, in consultation with the oncologist, we emphasize the unavoidability of the melanoma unit in the management of melanoma, since even before we are in stage III, the patient can be offered the possibility of immunotherapy that guarantees a statistically significant improvement of relapse-free survival (RFS), reducing the risk of disease recurrence or death [20]. Today we know that the choice of sending a patient to perform a biopsy of the sentinel lymph node is no longer solely guided by the thickness greater than or equal to 0.8 mm or the presence or absence of ulceration, and so it is essential to take into account all the aspects with which pathologists enrich our reports, aspects such as mitosis, index of replicative activity Ki67, lymphocytic infiltrates peritumoral (TILs), regression, vascular invasion, and perineural infiltration, which are a valuable guide in our therapeutic conduct [21].

## 4. Conclusions

With increasing incidence rates in all age categories and geographical areas, skin cancer is still a major worldwide health issue in 2024. The epidemiological trends for melanoma and non-melanoma skin cancers have been described in this chapter, with special emphasis on the intricate interactions between socioeconomic, environmental, and genetic factors that affect risk. Results are nevertheless influenced by regional differences, especially in access to healthcare; although some nations with high incidence rates benefit from early detection initiatives and cutting-edge therapies, others have disproportionately high fatality rates. Reducing the worldwide incidence of skin cancer and enhancing patient outcomes require sustained investment in preventive measures, enhanced diagnostic technologies, and fair access to therapy.

## Conflict of interest

The authors declare no conflict of interest.

## Notes/thanks/other declarations

None.

## Author details

Serena Federico[1], Francesco Fortarezza[2], Giuseppe Ingravallo[3] and Gerardo Cazzato[3]*

1 Dermatology Unit, University Hospital Renato Dulbecco, Magna Graecia University, Catanzaro, Italy

2 Surgical Pathology and Cytopathology Unit, University Hospital of Padova, Padova, Italy

3 Section of Molecular Pathology, Department of Precision and Regenerative Medicine and Ionian Area (DiMePRe-J), University of Bari "Aldo Moro", Bari, Italy

*Address all correspondence to: gerardo.cazzato@uniba.it

## References

[1] Narayanan DL, Saladi RN, Fox JL. Review: Ultraviolet radiation and skin cancer. International Journal of Dermatology. 2010;**49**(9):978-986

[2] Leiter U, Keim U, Garbe C. Epidemiology of skin cancer: Update 2019. Advances in Experimental Medicine and Biology. 2020;**1268**:123-139. DOI: 10.1007/978-3-030-46227-7_6

[3] Rogers HW, Weinstock MA, Harris AR, Hinckley MR, Feldman SR, Fleischer AB, et al. Incidence estimate of nonmelanoma skin cancer in the United States, 2006. Archives of Dermatology. 2010;**146**(3):283-287. DOI: 10.1001/archdermatol.2010.19

[4] Kim DP, Kus KJB, Ruiz E. Basal cell carcinoma review. Hematology/Oncology Clinics of North America. 2019;**33**(1): 13-24. DOI: 10.1016/j.hoc.2018.09.004

[5] Muzic JG, Schmitt AR, Wright AC, et al. Incidence and trends of basal cell carcinoma and cutaneous squamous cell carcinoma: A population-based study in Olmsted County, Minnesota, 2000 to 2010. Mayo Clinic Proceedings. 2017;**92**(6):890-898. DOI: 10.1016/j.mayocp.2017.02.015

[6] Canadian Cancer Statistics Advisory Committee. Canadian Cancer Statistics 2019. Toronto, ON: Canadian Cancer Society; 2019

[7] Madan V, Lear JT, Szeimies RM. Non-melanoma skin cancer. Lancet. 2010;**375**(9715):673-685

[8] John SM, Trakatelli M, Gehring R, Finlay K, Fionda C, Wittlich M, et al. CONSENSUS REPORT: Recognizing non-melanoma skin cancer, including actinic keratosis, as an occupational disease - a call to action. Journal of the European Academy of Dermatology and Venereology. 2016;**30**(Suppl 3):38-45. DOI: 10.1111/jdv.13608

[9] Cancer Research UK. Available from: https://www.cancerresearchuk.org/health-professional/cancer-statistics/statistics-by-cancer-type/non-melanoma-skin-cancer/incidence [Accessed: 10, 2024]

[10] Staples MP, Elwood M, Burton RC, Williams JL, Marks R, Giles GG. Non-melanoma skin cancer in Australia: The 2002 national survey and trends since 1985. The Medical Journal of Australia. 2006;**184**(1):6-10

[11] Sunsmart Australia. SunSmart campaign. Melbourne: Cancer Council Victoria; 2015

[12] Iwasaki M, Tsugane S. Risk factors for non-melanoma skin cancer in Japanese populations. Journal of Epidemiology. 2017;**17**(2):30-36

[13] Raman V, Satyanarayana D, Prakash P. Arsenic exposure and risk of squamous cell carcinoma: A review. Dermatologic Clinics. 2016;**34**(2):193-202

[14] Ezenwa E et al. Skin cancer and its implications in sub-Saharan Africa: A review. Nigerian Medical Journal. 2018;**59**(3):174-182

[15] Arnold M, Singh D, Laversanne M, Vignat J, Vaccarella S, Meheus F, et al. Global burden of cutaneous melanoma in 2020 and projections to 2040. JAMA Dermatology. 2022;**158**(5):495-503. DOI: 10.1001/jamadermatol.2022.0160

[16] Tímár J, Ladányi A. Molecular pathology of skin melanoma:

Epidemiology, differential diagnostics, prognosis and therapy prediction. International Journal of Molecular Sciences. 2022;**23**(10):5384. DOI: 10.3390/ijms23105384

[17] Bray F, Laversanne M, Sung H, Ferlay J, Siegel RL, Soerjomataram I, et al. Global cancer statistics 2022: GLOBOCAN estimates of incidence and mortality worldwide for 36 cancers in 185 countries. CA: a Cancer Journal for Clinicians. 2024;**74**(3):229-263. DOI: 10.3322/caac.21834. Epub 2024 Apr 4

[18] Ferrara G, Argenziano G. The WHO 2018 classification of cutaneous melanocytic neoplasms: Suggestions from routine practice. Frontiers in Oncology. 2021;**11**:675296. DOI: 10.3389/fonc.2021.675296

[19] Brancaccio G, Russo T, Lallas A, Moscarella E, Agozzino M, Argenziano G. Melanoma: clinical and dermoscopic diagnosis. Giornale Italiano di Dermatologia e Venereologia. 2017;**152**(3):213-223. DOI: 10.23736/S0392-0488.17.05571-7. Epub 2017 Jan 24

[20] Luke JJ, Rutkowski P, Queirolo P, Del Vecchio M, Mackiewicz J, Chiarion-Sileni V, et al. Pembrolizumab versus placebo as adjuvant therapy in completely resected stage IIB or IIC melanoma (KEYNOTE-716): A randomised, double-blind, phase 3 trial. Lancet. 2022;**399**(10336):1718-1729. DOI: 10.1016/S0140-6736(22)00562-1. Epub 2022 Apr 1

[21] Weyers W. The 'epidemic' of melanoma between under- and overdiagnosis. Journal of Cutaneous Pathology. 2012;**39**(1):9-16. DOI: 10.1111/j.1600-0560.2011.01831.x

Section 2

# Basal Cell Carcinoma (BCC)

Chapter 3

# Basal Cell Carcinoma

*Muhammad Salman Khalid, Muhammad Ammad Jamil, Adeeb Shehzad, Somia Mazhar and Farhan Hameed*

## Abstract

Globally, Basal cell carcinoma is the most prevalent form of skin cancer, which originates from basal cells of the epidermis. Sun-exposed parts of the body (head, face, and neck) are mostly affected by BCC. Characteristics of BCC include local invasiveness, low potential of metastasis, and slow growth. Despite its relatively low rate of mortality, it presents a significant public health concern, as its incidence rate is continuously rising. Different factors like aging population, sun-exposure, and behavior changes in lifestyle plays an important role in increasing BCC incident rate. UV exposure remains the dominant factor, immunosuppression, environmental influences, and genetic susceptibility also play important roles in amplifying the impact of UV on the skin. Different signaling pathways are involved in BCC pathogenesis which leads to tumor formation and cell proliferation. Targeting these pathways could lead to new diagnostic tools and treatment therapies. Clinically, there are different subtypes of BCC with unique features, morphologies, and characteristics. After early detection through visual inspection, Dermascopy, biopsy, and confocal microscopy techniques are used to diagnose BCC. Available treatment options include surgical excision. Cryosurgery, Mohs micrographic surgery, photodynamic therapy (PDT), radiotherapy, curettage and electrodessication therapy, and targeted molecular therapies.

**Keywords:** basal cell carcinoma, pathophysiology, cancer genetics, hedgehog pathway, prognosis

## 1. Introduction

Basal cell carcinoma (previously called basal cell epithelioma), is regarded as the most common and frequently occurring type of skin cancer worldwide, comprising about 80% of all cases of skin cancer. This specific type of cancer arises in the basal cells of the skin, which are the deepest layer of the cells in the epidermis [1]. The clinical presentation can be highly variable, from isolated erythematous/pigmented patch to papule, nodule, or ulcer of red-colored spots on different areas of the skin, including the scalp, face, and sometimes extremities. Although the rate at which it spreads is lower than the two other types, it can very rarely metastasize to other organs. Most of the time, it is associated with damage to DNA caused by ultraviolet radiation from the sun, and without any proper care, it can metastasize to other organs (in some of rare cases), but if left untreated it can cause serious implications [2].

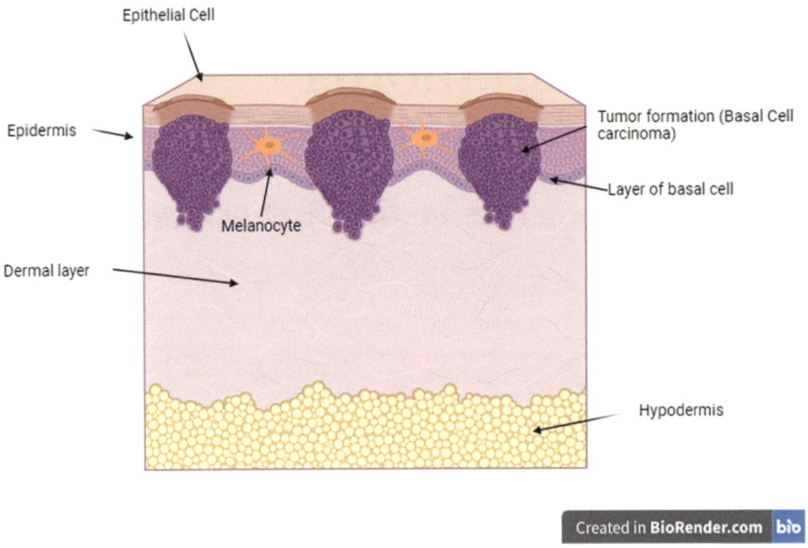


**Figure 1.**
*Generalized overview of the formation and progression of BCC in the basal cells of the skin. The formation of these sorts of tumors is promoted by exposure to UV radiation, the most common etiological factor in the development of BCC, ultimately leading toward the uncontrolled growth of the cells [6].*

According to reported literature, there are almost 26 different subtypes of skin cancer, from which the most reoccurring are micronodular, superficial, nodular, infiltrative, morpheaform, and fibroepithelioma of Pinkus (fibroepithelial skin cancer). Sometimes these subtypes can appear in a groups of 2–3 [3]. Clinical examination of BCC shows pink-colored cells with telangiectatic vessels (malformation of blood vessels). Treatment strategy for BCC includes surgical excision, Cryosurgery, Electrodesiccation, and Mohs surgery, and these treatments are good for localized BCC (shows more than 95% cure rate).

Exposure to Ultra-Violet (UV) rays is by far the most reported factor throughout the literature. Mostly UV-B radiations are associated with the development of BCC, but UV-A can also cause the predisposition to mutations in normal basal cells. The rate of incidence is typically higher in males than females due to more sun-exposure, but with the passage of time, this gender-related difference is becoming less significant as lifestyles of females changed considerably (use of tanning bed or smoking) [4]. Workers are at greater risk of BCC due to frequent accumulation of UV-rays, and the Fritzpatrick scale is quite often used for the prediction of skin cancer, usually white individuals are at a greater risk [5]. Types of skin and the exposure to ultraviolet rays are not the only predictors; the intensity of rays combined with the duration of exposure (mainly in childhood) plays a crucial role in the development of BCC (**Figure 1**).

## 2. Epidemiology

The incidence rate of BCC is rising at an alarming rate worldwide, and males are mostly affected by this type of cancer than females. The rate of incidence is also based on geographical regions and those regions which have lower or higher attitudes.

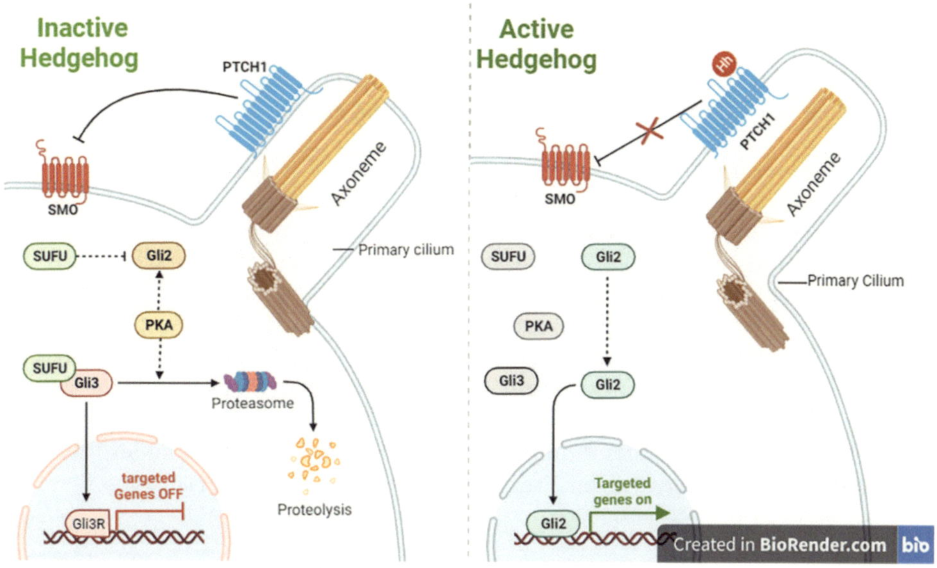


**Figure 2.**
*Generalized overview of the Hedgehog pathway in the activation of transcription factors. In the absence of the ligand (Hh), Smo is inhibited by the PTCH1 and Gli 3 is degraded by the proteasome system and targeted genes were not activated (Left). However, in the presence of the ligand, Smo is activated and PKA does not phosphorylate the Gli 2, which then translocates into the nucleus and causes the activation of transcription factors (Right) [13].*

A previous history of BCC is one of the best predictors of the development of this skin cancer, and according to recently published data, people with previous exposure to this disease are at a greater risk of developing BCC again compared to those patients who do not have such history [7]. According to data published over the last 25 years, the rate of incidence has increased to approximately 45%, and it is intricately linked with age (age more than 50 years). The mortality rate is preferably lower than the other two main types of skin tumors, and mostly patients with a weakened immune system are at risk. Tumors that show aggressive patterns in histopathological analysis are the common cause of metastasis, and if a tumor does metastasize, it usually invades lymph nodes, lungs, bones along with the skin [7].

The rate of incidence of Basal cell carcinoma in different races is given below, and most of the people affected by this cancer are Hispanics, Caucasians, Japanese and Chinese Asians [8–10]. Among different ethnicities, the incidence rate in Blacks is comparatively lower than the other (1–2 per million), and Africans residents have the lowest rate (0.065 per million). On the contrary, Chinese men and women are at a greater risk of developing this cancer, with 6.4 and 5.8 cases per million in men and women respectively. Furthermore, the prevalence of BCC is much higher in residents of Okinawa and Kawaii, with the rate of incidence reaching almost 30% [11]. Contrary to this, it is highly prevalent in Asian Indians and Blacks, and there are rare chances of this type to occur in Blacks, while most of the time, Whites are more affected [12]. According to data collected from different medical centers, the prevalence of Basal cell carcinoma accounts for 2–3% of the total annual cases [8]. The **Figure 2** shows cancer on different skin types [14]. The incidence of this cancer is highly dependent on the age factor and advances with the increase in age and approximately 40% of the patients that are diagnosed with this disease develop more lesions within the next 4–6 years [2, 15].

## 3. Etiology

Several factors (Genetic, Environmental) participate in the progression and development of BCC and all of those are summarized below:

### 3.1 Environmental factors

Environmental factors are among the fundamental and mostly analyzed risk factors in the study of basal cell carcinoma. Among these, exposure to UV light is the leading cause of the development of this disease (both UV-A and UV-B radiations are responsible). Too much exposure to these radiations causes the disruptions in the Deoxyribonucleic acid (DNA) that lead to mutations in the pro-oncogenes (that are close to developing cancer) and tumor suppressor genes (that controls the rate of mutations and protects the genome), and this in turn leads to the development of Basal cell carcinoma [7]. Other dominant factors are ionizing rays, includes gamma and X-rays, and exposure to arsenic further increases the risk of this disease.

### 3.2 Genetic factors

Genetic factors also play a key role in basal cell carcinoma progression and invasion. Mostly, mutations are seen in the sonic hedgehog pathway (SHH). This pathway performs a crucial role in developmental biology, responsible for cells differentiation in complex multicellular organisms (the pathway itself contains a series of complex interconnected molecules). The main proteins involved in this pathway are the transmembrane protein known as patched (Ptch) and another protein called smoothened (Smo). Smoothened is restricted by the patched protein, and the degradation of Ptch lead to the activation of Smo, which in turns favors the activation of Gli (Glioma associated oncogene transcription factor) that are involved in the activation of genes that controls cell growth and development [16].

Other dominant mutation is seen in Gorlin's syndrome (another name used for basal cell nevus syndrome [BCNS]), caused by mutations in the PTCH1 gene. This syndrome is closely linked with the progression and development of a lot of BCCs at early age, and the key characteristic abnormalities of this syndrome are ectopic calcifications, jaw cysts, and plantar. The PTCH1 gene participates in the suppression of tumors in the genome, and a loss of function is associated with the progression of Gorlin's syndrome [17].

### 3.3 Individual susceptibility factors

Several individuals also contributes toward the pathogenesis of basal cell carcinoma, including immunosuppression (those people who have weak immune system or those with disease like AIDS (acquired immune deficiency syndrome) are at a greater risk of developing BCC), type of skin (dark colored individuals are protected from BCC than light colored and fair colored skin due to large concentrations of melanin produced by the melanocytes), age (people with increasing age, greater than 50 years, are at a risk of developing bcc).

## 4. Pathophysiology of BCC

Excessive sunlight exposure appears as the primary risk factor contributing to BCC. Direct DNA damage is responsible for the development of basal cell carcinoma, accompanied by indirect damage to the DNA through the suppression of the immune system and ROS [4, 18]. Melanin also plays a role in indirect damage by absorbing UV-A radiation, and causes damage to DNA, while UV-B is responsible for direct damage to RNA (ribonucleic acid) and DNA with a transition of the CC/TT [4]. Exposure to ultraviolet radiation also causes immune suppression of cutaneous cells, leading to the dysregulation of the immune system. According to studies published in the near past, BCC arises in those cells that are immature or are transiting from the immature to mature stage, cells related to hair follicles. One of the key genes dysregulated in BCC is PTCH1, and mutation in this gene is associated with 70% of the cases of BCC, while 20% of the patients of this type depicts the mutation the SMO gene. The inactivation of the PTCH1 or the high expressions of the Gli, by the trans activation of the smoothened is good enough to drive the progression of basal cell carcinoma. Second most vital dysregulation in basal cell carcinoma is the mutation in the gatekeeper gene P53 [19, 20].

### 4.1 Canonical hedgehog pathway

The HH pathways participate in mitogenesis and division of cells, and this pathway is activated when hedgehog protein binds to its receptors, and activates interlinked pathways. Vertebrates consists of three main kinds of Hh proteins: Desert hedgehog (DHH), Sonic hedgehog (SHH), and Indian hedgehog (IHH), and all these three are involved in the activation of the same pathway but do so by activating several different genes [4]. The receptor for Shh is Ptch (a transmembrane protein), and after binding of Shh, the receptor is degraded by the proteosome system inside the cell. This degradation leads to the migration of Smo into membrane, and Gli family of proteins are activated, that translocates from the cell into the nucleus and there acts a transcription factor by modulating several key genes that are engaged in control of cell development. If the pathways are not functional, Gli proteins are phosphorylated (a phosphate group is added), and they become repressor Gli proteins. This Gli-R also translocates to nucleus but here causes the suppression of all those genes that takes part in the HH pathway and hence the amount of Gli to Gli-R inside the cell plays the most crucial role in governing that which genes are to be expressed and which are to be repressed [21].

Hyper-activation of the Hedgehog (HH) signaling pathway, corresponding to the canonical hedgehog, is the most common hallmark in studying the progression of basal cell carcinoma, as reported by various studies conducted in the past [22]. This pathway plays a vital role in cell differentiation, proliferation, and embryogenesis in the preliminary stages of cell development, this facilitates the development of epidermis by the crosstalk between dermal cells of the skin and those cells that are of epithelial origin. Canonical activation of the pathway is driven by ligands names as sonic hedgehog (SHH), Indian Hedgehog (IHH), and sometimes by Desert Hedgehog (DHH) in response of the PTCH1 receptor [23]. Activation of this pathway do facilitate the activation of this gene and this Smo migrates to one of the highly specialized primary cilia and as a result, SMO drives the hyper-activation of the Gli transcription factors followed by the suppression of the fused (SUFU- suppressor of fused homolog). However, if HH does not attach to PTCH1, the Gli family of transcription factors are in their inactive form as Smo does not translocate to the primary cilia and the Gli proteins are ubiquitinated [24, 25]. The eventual results from the activation of this signaling cascade is dependent on differentiation and proliferation, self-renewal, cell survival (by the activation of the BCL-2 (B-cell lymphoma −2) protein family), transition from epithelium to mesenchymal cells, angiogenesis, and invasiveness of BCC.

### 4.2 Non-canonical hedgehog

However, in the case of non-canonical signaling, HH interacts with a lot of other signaling networks that are oncogenic in nature, such as IGF, TGFβ, aPKC, NF-kB, and epidermal growth factor receptor (EGFR). These pathways synergistically contribute to the progression of basal cell carcinoma. It means that, the activation of the Gli family of receptors may be done by many alternative pathways that are non-canonical, but all this happens in the absence of bypassing Smo [26, 27]. The activity of Gli is positively influenced by the RAS, PI3K, and AKT, while it is negatively regulated by the P53 family of proteins and significantly the expression of the RAS/RAF cascade, which further hyper-activates the JUN complex, causing the progression of developmental processes. TGF-beta signaling do activates the upregulation of GLI2 transcription, while GLI1 is activated by the complex protein, aPKC [28]. Furthermore, IGF-1 causes the induction of the nuclear localization of GLI1 and 2, and it has also been observed that the activation of PI3K and AKT regulates epithelial-mesenchymal transformation and the secretion of matrix metalloproteinases (MMP's) [29]. The **Figure 3** shows the dysregulation in the non-canonical pathway.

### 4.3 Other genetic alterations

Apart from alterations in hedgehog pathway, several other genetic changes have also been reported in the literature that contribute toward the pathogenesis of basal cell carcinoma, and these alterations do not depend on the activation of the HH

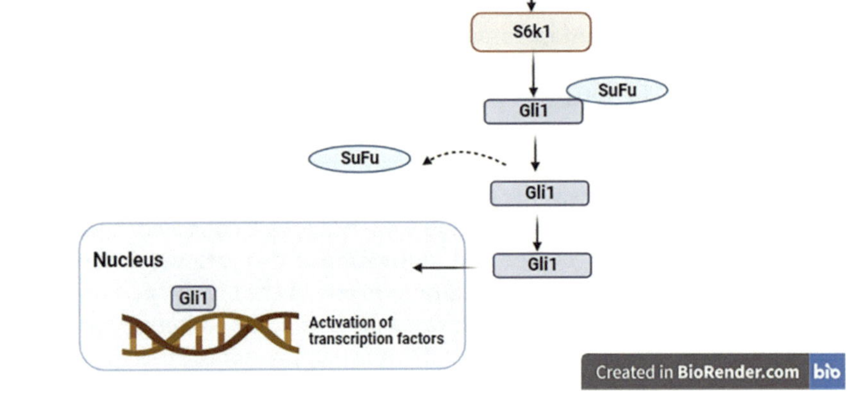


**Figure 3.**
*Non-canonical Hedgehog pathway mediated by the phosphorylation of AKT, TSC22, and S6K1 instead of the attachement of Hh ligand. The phosphorylation of AKT by PI3K mediates the activation of the Gli family of transcription factors. Phosphorylation of S6k1 enzyme is facilitated by the inhibition of mTOR which then activates the Gli family of protein in by the help of SuFu gene. Phosphorylation of this Gli allows it to translocates from cytoplasm to the nucleus and causes the activation of potential genes [30].*

pathway. These includes dysregulation in the Hippo-Yap and WNT signaling (Hippo pathway is associated with the controlled growth of organs and WNT signaling pathway is associated with development of embryo) pathways. The main effector protein that is altered is the Yes-associated protein (YAP), which participates in maintaining progenitors and proliferation of the skin and upon its phosphorylation it translocates in cytoplasm, thus being unable to transcribe the associated genes [31]. While in case of WNT signaling, several changes have been observed in the activation of downstream effectors as well as the destruction of β-catenin (after the phosphorylation of disheveled and inhibition of GSK-3β). Dysregulation in this pathway is typically due to the activation of WNT by the Gli proteins, which lead to the upregulation of several stem cells markers [32].

Missense mutation in the N-Myc gene also contributes to the basal cell carcinoma progression (Myc transcription factors are responsible for cell growth, proliferation, and development of embryo) because it is one of the downstream effectors of HH signaling. Most of the time alteration arises when this gene interacts with the tumor suppressor FBXW7 that is involved in the degradation of Myc (proteosome dependent destruction of MYC) [33, 34]. Mutations in NOTCH signaling have also been reported to play a part in the progression of BCC. It is one of the targets of the guardian gene, p53, and is responsible for epidermal differentiation. Although mutation in this gene is not regarded as the driver mutations but still these are the most common mutations in BCC [35].

## 5. Histopathology and subtyping

The clusters of basaloid cells form the islands which exhibit the distinct appearance characteristic of BCCs. In BCCs formation, irregular arrangement of basaloid cells can be seen in the center with a palisade arrangement at periphery. Each basaloid cell contains staining nucleus that lacks a visible nucleolus and contains marginal or limited cytoplasm. Upon examining the paraffin-embedded sections between the tumor and its stromal neighbors, a retraction artifact also known as clefting.

When examined on paraffin-embedded sections, a retraction artifact, identified as clefting. Additionally, mucin deposition is also present within the tumor and its neighboring tissue. The aggressive form of disease can be indicated by the existence of perineural growth [7, 36].

Trichoblastoma and trichoepithelioma are the conditions involved in the histological differential diagnosis. Many different structural subtypes have been identified i.e., superficial, infiltrating, nodular, micronodular, pigmented, sclerosing, fibroepitheliomatous etc. In mixed patterns, combinations of above listed types were observed.

- Superficial subtypes comprise of multiple basaloid cells which are small, that extend from epidermis but do not penetrate in the dermis.

- Most cases are associated with modular type. Nodular basal cell carcinomas consist of clusters of cells which display outer lining and irregular arrangement in their central region. Ulceration can be seen in larger lesions.

- The micronodular subtype's histological characteristics resemble nodular subtypes characteristics. Micronodular subtypes contain many nodular, which make it different from nodular subtype. For local recurrence, micronodular subtype has greater risk than solid type.

- Sclerosing subtype morphology contains thin strands of basaloid and spiky cells which are surrounded by thick fibrous stroma that invade the dermis. It is challenging to histological differentiate this from conditions like, metastatic cancer, microcystic adnexal carcinoma, or desmoplastic trichoepithelioma. The term infiltrative BCCs is used when tumor nests have spiky projections which invade deeply [37].

- Combination of melanocytes and melanin results in the pigmented BCCs. This phenomenon is mostly seen in variations of micronodular, superficial, and follicular.

- Infundibulocystic variation forms compact, and well-defined tumor consists of clusters of cells with interconnecting pattern arrangement with minimal stroma. This variation is not common and mostly found on the face. Melanin and keratinous matter are present in structure of many small infundibular cysts.

- Soft, nodular lesions are present fibroepithelioma of Pinkus, which resembles papilloma and fibroma. This subtype is often found on the lower back. Structurally it is composed of a grouping of basaloid cells and interconnected strands which are surrounded by fibrous stroma [36, 37].

## 6. Diagnosis

The diverse pathological presentation of basal cell carcinoma consists of many subtypes, such as nodular, fibroepithelial, superficial, and infiltrative BCC, each exhibiting distinct clinicopathological characteristics. Additionally, micronodular subtypes hold significant histopathological relevance with the basosquamous subtype which impacts both prognosis of patient and approaches of treatment. Furthermore, multiple tumor subtypes display histopathological of features within the same lesion. Dermascopy is most useful in the diagnosis of basal cell carcinoma and differentiation of non-pigmented BCC from pigmented ones. This is characterized by the development of arborizing vessels and globules of blue-gray colors with a leaf like structure. The differential diagnosis is sometimes confused with the diffusion of trichoepithelioma, while superficial basal cell carcinoma could mimic some inflammatory conditions like eczema and psoriasis [38].

Apart from dermascopy, some novel diagnostic approaches are also practiced worldwide, and these techniques provide a clearer picture about the diagnosis of BCC based on its different subtypes. These techniques include optical coherence tomography (OCT), Raman spectroscopy (RS), multiphoton tomography (MPS), and confocal laser scanning microscopy (CLSM).

### 6.1 Optical coherence tomography

it is a noninvasive imaging technique that provides the cross-sectional interpretation of tissues that helps in visualizing the structure of epidermis and papillary dermis up to depth of approximately 2 mm. It uses low length of coherence light as a source to visualize the skin structures properties. OCT also provides the visual characteristics of superficial and dermal tumor nests. Therefore, it is also used in differentiation of different subtypes of BCC.

### 6.2 Raman spectroscopy

Raman spectroscopy imaging provides quantitative view of structure. Light of infrared wavelength is used to differentiate different cutaneous structures. Different energy vibrations are generated by each structure when light is scattered on them. These vibrations of energy resemble their spectral peak, which is detected by meter, providing a quantitative view. Raman spectroscopy can be used to detect cellular alteration caused due to cancerous tumors. Generally, Raman spectroscopy is time consuming technique, therefore, to overcome this issue other modalities have been used by researchers.

### 6.3 Multiphoton spectroscopy

Multiphoton spectroscopy is used *in vivo* for dermatologic purposes. In this technique, fluorescence is excited from the target through simulating the two or more infrared light photons absorption. Then raster-scanning is used to generate the images. MPS has a spatial lateral resolution of 1 mm and a spatial axial resolution of 2 mm. Fluorescence lifetime imaging microscopy (FLIM) is used to differentiate between the corresponding tissue and fluorescence. It measures the decaying rate of the fluorescence signal and short excited pulse follows. For detection of BCC from normal skin cells multispectral FLIM multiphoton tomography is used [39].

### 6.4 Confocal laser scanning microscopy

Confocal laser scanning uses fluorescence or reflectance modes. Reflectance confocal microscopy (RCM) is used *in vivo* to produce real-time 2D horizontal image. Cellular resolution from the epidermis to papillary dermal layers can be produced from it. CLSM has a lateral resolution of 250 nm and a depth of 1 μm. The CLSM mechanism involves the laser source with a specific wavelength. This light visualizes the tissue within the skin after its transmission. After transmission, the light is reflected and passes through the pinhole in the optical conjugate plane. In the detector, a 2D image is formed. On the other hand, RCM images depend on reflectivity differences within normal and cancer tissues. High refractive index structures appear bright in images [40].

## 7. Treatment

As there is not much risk of metastasis in BCC, treatment for primary lesions is easy and that is why chances of fighting against it are very high. Although there are many established and well-designed therapies against it, the health of patients is the primary concern before choosing an appropriate method (condition of patient as well as recurrence of disease should be kept in mind) [34, 41]. Certain etiological factors associated with it are prior exposure to radiotherapy, poor border clarity, weakened immune system, and a recurrent tumor. Before choosing an appropriate method of treatment, a biopsy should be done to gain information about the prevalent subtype of BCC, and the following things are kept in mind while treating this condition [42].

- Complete removal of lesions to prevent the reappearance.
- Correction of any impairment that results from the lesions.
- Providing patients with the best cosmetics because most of the time BCC is diagnosed on the face.

BCC is mostly treated by surgical excision, but in some cases, it can be treated with chemotherapy as well as radiotherapy. Some of the most common treatment options are described below:

### 7.1 Surgical excision

Surgical excision is regarded as the standard treatment for BCC as it is highly effective and can remove all the lesions (having cure rate of more than 96%). In this technique, clinicians remove the lesions with a sharp object (some healthy cells are also removed that are near the cancerous lesions). After that, margins are analyzed with the help of microscope to confirm that there are no other cancerous cells remaining. Although considered the most effective and easiest way mode of treatment, the results of this treatment are scars that are white in color.

### 7.2 Mohs micrographic surgery

This technique is regarded as the gold standard for the treatment of high-risk basal cell carcinoma and is the only current option that provides a long-term cure with the potential advantage of tissue sparing. This treatment option allows accurate evaluation of the margins of the lesions, the lesions (tumors) are cut out layer by layer and microscopic evaluation of each layer is done on the spot. High rate of cure is associated with 100% accurate examination as compared to other techniques that only examine less than 1% of margins. This helps in only taking those areas where there is positive tumor by minimizing the size of wound [43].

### 7.3 Radiotherapy

Radiotherapy is another considerable option for the treatment of BCC if surgery is not recommended. This technique is also applicable for the treatment of cancerous lesions when further surgical excision could result in the loss of major nerves or crucial structures. The cure rate of radiotherapy is almost 93%, but the appearance of BCC after this treatment can be aggressive than the previous one and this technique also has some side effects that appear after sometimes, including fibrosis of dermal tissues, alopecia, inflammation of the skin, and necrosis. Based on these outcomes, radiotherapy is generally used for those patients only who are not ready for surgical treatment (that have lesions in those areas associated with high-risk) [44].

### 7.4 Photodynamic therapy

Another treatment option is photodynamic therapy (PDT), which uses a focused beam of light on the lesions for many hours after treating the skin with photosensitizing porphyrins like methyl aminolevulinate (MAL). Tumors are destroyed when reactive oxygen species, induced when photosensitizer absorbs light, cause cytotoxicity that helps in producing a local inflammatory response that aids in the destruction. Although the technique is less invasive, but still the cure rates vary (almost 87%) depending on the absorption capacity of the photosensitizer. BCC that are superficial in nature are more effectively treated among all the subtypes and is under practice in most of the European countries for effectively treating superficial BCC [45].

### 7.5 Imiquimod therapy

The drug imiquimod is an immune system modulator that is currently administered as a topical treatment in the US and Europe. It is used for the treatment of basal cell carcinoma in such patients that are immunocompetent. Its mechanism includes the production of proinflammatory cytokines after its binding to the specific toll-like receptors present on the cells, allowing it to induce cytotoxic T-cell mediated death of the cancerous cells [46]. The duration of this treatment is approximately 6 weeks, and the rate of cure is comparatively greater (83.4%) than that of photodynamic therapy (72.8%) and 5-flourouracil (80.1%). Furthermore, the probability of tumor free survival after a duration of 5 years was 80.5%, greater than the PDT and 5-flourouracil. Apart from its high cure rate, the main disadvantage of this medication is the inability to penetrate deeply in the skin (does not have any therapeutic effects on nodular tumors). This therapy is not recommended for such diseases that have the chances to re-appear, but is only suitable for such patients that prefer non-surgical mode of treatment [47].

### 7.6 Targeted therapy

Smo inhibitors are regarded as the prime method of treatment for metastatic and advanced BCC and these inhibitors include sonidegib and vismodegib (are orally administered and currently approved by the US Food and Drug administration (FDA) and European Medicines Agency (EMA)). Although they are good for controlling metastatic BCC, but these also have some side effects as loss of taste, hair loss, weight loss, and diarrhea [36].

### 7.7 Cryosurgery

It is considered as an effective technique for basal cell carcinoma treatment due to its cost benefit ratio and ease of use. In this procedure, lesions of BCC are destroyed by freeze-thaw cycles and the cure rate of this technique is approximately 96%. This technique has some drawbacks as it cannot do fine assessment of tumor margins and is only limited to those BCC that are superficial in origin (low-risk of metastasis) [4].

### 7.8 Electrodessication and curettage

This mode of treatment is primarily done for the management of low-risk BCC's and is also a cost- effective technique recommended by the National Comprehensive Cancer Network (NCCN). The procedure applied for the treatment is cutting off lesions with the help of curette and then burning those cancerous cells with an electric needle. The main consideration when using this is to avoid such areas that have hair growth on terminals, as there is a high chance of extension of tumors in those areas (pubis, scalp, and chin). Inadequate assessment of tumor margins is the main drawback of this technique [4].

## 8. Discussions

Emerging trends in the incidence of basal cell carcinoma (BCC) have been reported by recent epidemiological research. These patterns indicate a changing demographic landscape, with a growing frequency among younger individuals. This demographic shift highlights the need for increased awareness and focused preventative measures to combat the growing burden of BCC.

Understanding of the etiological elements, responsible for BCC development has improved because of advances in genetic and molecular studies. Mutations in hedgehog signaling pathway genes, such as SMO and PTCH1, have been found to be important cancer drivers. BCC pathogenesis is also influenced by interactions between genetic predisposition and environmental exposures, including UV radiation and immunological dysregulation. Targeted treatment strategies are made possible by the complex interactions among immune responses, tumor microenvironment, and genetic abnormalities in the pathophysiology of BCC. In advanced or metastatic BCC, new immunotherapeutic strategies, such as immune checkpoint inhibitors and targeted biologic agents, show promise for enhancing treatment results and lowering disease recurrence.

Technological developments in diagnostic modalities including a molecular profiling, reflectance confocal microscopy, and dermascopy have improved our ability to identify and categorize BCC subtypes. By making early detection, accurate tumor margin delineation, and knowledgeable treatment decision, these techniques improve outcomes and patient care. Regarding therapy, current clinical studies have investigated cutting-edge therapeutic approaches meant to get beyond resistance mechanisms and boost response rates in BCC cases that are refractory. For individuals with few therapeutic choices, targeted treatments such as hedgehog pathway inhibitors (like vismodegib and sonidegib) have shown a hope in treating advanced or metastatic BCC.

Additionally, attempts to maximize surgical methods, such as minimally invasive treatments and Mohs micrographic surgery, try to accomplish total tumor removal while maintaining esthetic results and reducing functional impact. In high-risk or recurring BCC instances, adjuvant treatments such photodynamic therapy and radiation are helpful supplements to surgery. To sum up, the discussion about basal cell carcinoma highlights how complex the illness is, covering a wide range of topics including pathophysiology, diagnostics, etiology, epidemiology, and therapies. Continual research projects and teamwork are crucial to expanding our knowledge of BCC and converting scientific findings into novel treatments that enhance patient outcomes and quality of life.

## 9. Conclusions

Regarded as the most prevalent type of skin cancer, mutations and alterations have been studied extensively. Although many genetic alterations are associated with the progression of this type of skin cancer, the main one is the dysregulation in the Hedgehog signaling pathway that enables it to originate in the basal cells of the skin, but rarely metastasize. Early diagnosis leads to controlled treatment options that are favorable for the patients as well as the health practitioners, and it also enables for the better clinical presentation of different subtypes of basal cell carcinoma based on their morphology and characteristics. Although available treatment options enable the clinicians to effectively neutralize it from the skin, but still, it can reoccur and most of the time, Moh's micrographic surgery and simple surgical excision provides the best cure rate. But recent advancements have enabled the researchers to identify potential molecules that drives BCC and based on these molecules a new approach has been in practice for the treatment of BCC; targeted therapy, that has increased the percentage of cure rate of the disease.

## Acknowledgements

I would like to thank my co-author, Muhammad Ammad Jamil, and supervisor, Dr. Adeeb Shehzad, from National University of Sciences and Technology (NUST), Islamabad for their assistance and help in writing this chapter.

## Conflicts of interest

The authors declare no conflict of interests in relation to this chapter.

## Appendices and nomenclature

| | |
|---|---|
| BCC | basal cell carcinoma |
| UV-rays | ultra-violet rays |
| DNA | deoxyribonucleic acid |
| Smo | smoothened |
| SHH | sonic hedgehog |
| Ptch | patched |
| BCNS | basal cell nevus syndrome |
| Gli | glioma associated oncogene transcription factor |
| AIDS | acquired immune deficiency syndrome |
| RNA | ribonucleic acid |
| DHH | desert hedgehog |
| IHH | Indian hedgehog |
| SUFU | suppressor of fused homolog |
| BCL-2 | B-cell lymphoma-2 |
| EGFR | epidermal growth factor receptor |
| MMP's | matrix metalloproteinases |
| YAP | yes-associated proteins |
| OCT | optical coherence tomography |
| RS | Raman spectroscopy |
| CLSM | confocal laser scanning microscopy |
| MPS | multiphoton spectroscopy |
| PDT | photodynamic therapy |
| FLIM | fluorescence lifetime imaging microscopy |
| RCM | reflectance confocal microscopy |
| MAL | methyl aminolevulinate |
| FDA | food and drug administration |
| EMA | European medicine agency |
| NCCN | national comprehensive cancer network |

## Author details

Muhammad Salman Khalid[1], Muhammad Ammad Jamil[1], Adeeb Shehzad[2]*, Somia Mazhar[1] and Farhan Hameed[1]

1 Department of Biomedical Engineering and Sciences, School of Mechanical and Manufacturing Engineering (SMME), National University of Sciences and Technology (NUST) Islamabad, Pakistan

2 Biodiversity Unit, Research Center, Dhofar University, Salalah, Oman

*Address all correspondence to: adeeb.shehzad@gmail.com

## References

[1] Qadir MI. Skin cancer: Etiology and management. Pakistan Journal of Pharmaceutical Sciences. 2016;**29**(3):999-1003

[2] Linares MA, Zakaria A, Nizran P. Skin cancer. Journal of Primary Care & Community Health. 2015;**42**(4):645-659

[3] Dai J et al. Identification of critically carcinogenesis-related genes in basal cell carcinoma. OncoTargets and Therapy. 2018;**11**:6957-6967. Published Online: 15 Oct 2018

[4] Fania L et al. Basal cell carcinoma: From pathophysiology to novel therapeutic approaches. Biomedicine. 2020;**8**(11):449

[5] Martens MC et al. Photocarcinogenesis and skin cancer prevention strategies: An update. Anticancer Research. 2018;**38**(2):1153-1158

[6] Teng Y, Yu Y, Li S, Huang Y, Xu D, Tao X, et al. Ultraviolet radiation and basal cell carcinoma: An environmental perspective. Frontiers in Public Health. 2021;**9**:666528

[7] Cameron MC et al. Basal cell carcinoma: Epidemiology; pathophysiology; clinical and histological subtypes; and disease associations. In: Part of the Book Series: Recent Results in Cancer Research. Conference Paper. Vol. 139. 2019. pp. 263-273

[8] Scotto J, Fears TR, Fraumeni JF. Incidence of nonmelanoma skin cancer in the United States. Bethesda, MD: U.S. Dept. of Health and Human Services, National Institutes of Health; 1983

[9] Koh D et al. Basal cell carcinoma, squamous cell carcinoma and melanoma of the skin: Analysis of the Singapore Cancer Registry data 1968-97. British Journal of Dermatology. 1 June 2003;**148**(6):1161-1166. DOI: 10.1046/j.1365-2133.2003.05223.x

[10] Ichihashi M et al. Trends in nonmelanoma skin cancer in Japan. In: Skin Cancer: Basic Science, Clinical Research and Treatment. Recent Results in Cancer Research. Vol. 139. Berlin, Heidelberg: Springer Verlag; 1995

[11] Munyao TM, Othieno-Abinya NA. Cutaneous basal cell carcinoma in Kenya. East African Medical Journal. 1 Feb 1999;**76**(2):97-100. PMID: 10442131

[12] Lesher JL Jr, d'Aubermont PC, Brown VM. Morpheaform basal cell carcinoma in a young black woman. The Journal of Dermatologic Surgery and Oncology. February 1988;**14**(2):200-203. DOI: 10.1111/j.1524-4725.1988.tb03363.x

[13] Basset-Seguin N, Herms FJAD-V. Update on the management of basal cell carcinoma. Acta Dermato-Venereologica. 2020;**100**(11)

[14] Eisemann N et al. Non-melanoma skin cancer incidence and impact of skin cancer screening on incidence. Journal of Investigative Dermatology. January 2014;**134**(1):43-50

[15] Gloster HM Jr, Neal K. Skin cancer in skin of color. Journal of the American Academy of Dermatology. November 2006;**55**(5):741-760

[16] Gutzmer R, Solomon JAJTO. Hedgehog pathway inhibition for the treatment of basal cell carcinoma. Targeted Oncology. 2019;**14**:253-267. Published: 26 June 2019

[17] Flowers L, Sandhu M, Martin K. Skin cancer: Basal cell nevus syndrome

(Gorlin syndrome). Journal of the Dermatology Nurses' Association. 2023;**15**(6):268-272. DOI: 10.1097/JDN.0000000000000764

[18] Jee BA et al. Molecular classification of basal cell carcinoma of skin by gene expression profiling. Molecular Carcinogenesis. December 2015;**54**(12):1605-1612

[19] Apalla Z et al. Skin cancer: Epidemiology, disease burden, pathophysiology, diagnosis, and therapeutic approaches. Dermatology and Therapy Review. 2017;7:5-19. Published: 1 February 2017

[20] Chamcheu JC et al. Role and therapeutic targeting of the PI3K/Akt/mTOR signaling pathway in skin cancer: A review of current status and future trends on natural and synthetic agents therapy. Cells. 2019;**8**(8):803. DOI: 10.3390/cells8080803

[21] Bakshi A et al. Basal cell carcinoma pathogenesis and therapy involving hedgehog signaling and beyond. Molecular Carcinogenesis. December 2017;**56**(12):2543-2557

[22] Epstein EH. Basal cell carcinomas: Attack of the hedgehog. Nature Reviews Cancer. 2008;**8**:743-754

[23] Adnan M et al. Exploring nanocarriers as treatment modalities for skin cancer. Molecules. 2023;**28**(15):5905. DOI: 10.3390/molecules28155905

[24] Pellegrini C et al. Understanding the molecular genetics of basal cell carcinoma. International Journal of Molecular Sciences. 2017;**18**(11):2485. DOI: 10.3390/ijms18112485

[25] Shehzad A. Cancer Biomarkers in Diagnosis and Therapeutics. Singapore: Springer; 2022

[26] Xu Z et al. Computer-aided diagnosis of skin cancer based on soft computing techniques. Open Medicine. 2020;**15**(1):860-871. DOI: 10.1515/med-2020-0131

[27] Shehzad A et al. Decursinol angelate inhibits PGE2-induced survival of the human leukemia HL-60 cell line via regulation of the EP2 receptor and NF κ B pathway. Cancer Biology and Therapy. 2016;**17**(9):985-993

[28] Rehman G et al. Role of AMP-activated protein kinase in cancer therapy. Archiv der Pharmazie. July 2014;**347**(7):457-468

[29] Yu C et al. Combination of immunotherapy with targeted therapy: Theory and practice in metastatic melanoma. Frontiers in Immunology. Sec. Cancer Immunity and Immunotherapy. 7 May 2019;**10**:990. DOI: 10.3389/fimmu.2019.00990

[30] Jenkins DJCS. Hedgehog signalling: Emerging evidence for non-canonical pathways. Cellular Signalling. 2009;**21**(7):1023-1034

[31] Furth N et al. p53 shades of hippo. Cell Death & Differentiation. 2018;**25**:81-92

[32] Carmon KS et al. LGR5 interacts and cointernalizes with Wnt receptors to modulate Wnt/β-catenin signaling. Molecular and Cellular Biology. 2012;**32**(11):2054-2064

[33] Hatton BA et al. N-myc is an essential downstream effector of Shh signaling during both normal and neoplastic cerebellar growth. Cancer Research. 2006;**66**(17):8655-8661. DOI: 10.1158/0008-5472.CAN-06-1621

[34] Hassan S et al. Diagnostic and therapeutic potential of circulating-free DNA and cell-free RNA in cancer management. Biomedicines.

2022;**10**(8):2047. DOI: 10.3390/biomedicines10082047

[35] Watt FM, Estrach S, Ambler CA. Epidermal Notch signalling: Differentiation, cancer and adhesion. Current Opinion in Cell Biology. April 2008;**20**(2):171-179

[36] Dika E et al. Basal cell carcinoma: A comprehensive review. International Journal of Molecular Sciences. 2020;**21**(15):5572. DOI: 10.3390/ijms21155572

[37] Kim DP, Kus KJB, Ruiz E. Basal cell carcinoma review. Hematology/Oncology Clinics of North America. 1 Feb 2019;**33**(1):13-24. DOI: 10.1016/j.hoc.2018.09.004

[38] Ghita MA et al. Reflectance confocal microscopy and dermoscopy for in vivo, non-invasive skin imaging of superficial basal cell carcinoma. Oncology Letters. May 2016;**11**(5):3019-3024. DOI: 10.3892/ol.2016.4354. Published Online on: March 21, 2016. Print ISSN: 1792-1074, Online ISSN:1792-1082

[39] Rossi AM et al. Novel approaches to imaging basal cell carcinoma. Future Oncology. 2015;**11**(12):3039-3046. Published Online: 15 Oct 2015

[40] Ilie MA et al. In vivo confocal laser scanning microscopy imaging of skin inflammation: Clinical applications and research directions. Experimental and Therapeutic Medicine. February 2019;**17**(2):1004-1011. DOI: 10.3892/etm.2018.6981. Published Online on: November 16, 2018. Print ISSN: 1792-0981, Online ISSN: 1792-1015

[41] Islam SU, Ahmed MB, Shehzad A, Lee YS. Methanolic extract of Artemia salina eggs and various fractions in different solvents contain potent compounds that decrease cell viability of colon and skin cancer cell lines and show antibacterial activity against Pseudomonas aeruginosa. Evidence Based Complementary and Alternative Medicine. 2019;**2019**:12. Article ID 9528256. DOI: 10.1155/2019/9528256

[42] Bichakjian CK et al. Basal cell skin cancer, version 1.2016, NCCN clinical practice guidelines in oncology. Journal of the National Comprehensive Cancer Network. May 2016;**14**(5):574-597. DOI: 10.6004/jnccn.2016.0065

[43] Rowe DE et al. Mohs surgery is the treatment of choice for recurrent (previously treated) basal cell carcinoma. The Journal of Dermatologic Surgery and Oncology. April 1989;**15**(4):424-431. DOI: 10.1111/j.1524-4725.1989.tb03249.x

[44] Fleming ID et al. Principles of management of basal and squamous cell carcinoma of the skin. Supplement: An Interdisciplinary International Journal of the American Cancer Society (Supplement). Cancer. 15 January 1995;**75**(S2):699-704

[45] Foley P. Clinical efficacy of methyl aminolevulinate (Metvix®) photodynamic therapy. Journal of Dermatological Treatment. 2003;**14**(sup3):15-22. Published Online: 18 Nov 2009

[46] Peris K et al. Diagnosis and treatment of basal cell carcinoma: European consensus–based interdisciplinary guidelines. European Journal of Cancer. September 2019;**118**:10-34

[47] Smith V, Walton S. Treatment of facial basal cell carcinoma: A review. Journal of Skin Cancer. 2011;**2011**:7. Article ID 380371. DOI: 10.1155/2011/380371

Chapter 4

# Multiple Basal Cell Carcinomas

*Qiaochu Zhou, Yanan Zhang, Shan Zhang, Jinhui Wang, Lele Lin and Jie Xu*

## Abstract

Basal cell carcinoma is a common nonmelanoma form of skin cancer. Treating multiple basal cell carcinomas is challenging, and choosing the best treatment for multiple basal cell carcinomas is a real problem for clinicians. The treatment of multiple basal cell carcinomas has seen a progressive evolution in recent years. Several tumor suppressor genes and proto-oncogenes have been implicated in BCC pathogenesis, including the key components of the Hedgehog pathway, PTCH1 and SMO, the TP53 tumor suppressor, and members of the RAS proto-oncogene family. A variety of treatment modalities exist and are selected. We reviewed the studies providing treatment options for multiple basal cell carcinomas. This review may be helpful to meet the challenges of management.

**Keywords:** basal cell carcinoma, multiple basal cell carcinomas, treatment option, Gorlin syndrome, Hedgehog pathway inhibitor, photodynamic therapy

## 1. Introduction

Basal cell carcinoma (BCC) is the most commonly diagnosed cancer and the most frequent skin cancer in the fair-skinned adult population of over 50 years of age. Globally, their incidence is on the rise [1]. The prognosis for basal cell carcinoma varies, from superficial or nodular lesions of good prognosis to very extensive, difficult-to-treat lesions that must be discussed in a multidisciplinary committee. The treatment and follow-up are depending on the type of BCC observed. There is a high risk in patients with multiple basal cell carcinomas. Treating multiple basal cell carcinomas is challenging, and choosing the best treatment for multiple basal cell carcinomas is a real problem for clinicians. The pathogenesis of BCC has been linked to a number of tumor suppressor genes and proto-oncogenes, including the key components of the Hedgehog pathway, PTCH1 and SMO, the TP53 tumor suppressor, and members of the RAS proto-oncogene family [2]. Recent years have witnessed a progressive evolution in treating multiple basal cell carcinoma following the introduction of inhibitors of the Hedgehog pathway.

## 2. Epidemiology

Basal cell carcinoma is the most common skin malignant tumor worldwide, especially in light-skinned people, and is more frequently seen in males.

The incidence of BCC ranges from 77 to 158 per 100,1000 patients in Europe and the lifetime risk of developing BCC is approximately 30% [3]. This number continues to increase annually over the last decades. Ultraviolet exposure is the major risk factor. As was reported, multiple BCCs were more frequently seen in old people and larger sizes in males [4]. B. Souto et al. indicated that 23.3% of patients had two or more BCCs, with an average age of 65 ± 15 years [5].

## 3. Risk factors and pathogenesis for multiple BCC

The risk for developing BCC can be due to constitutional predisposition (genotypic and phenotypic characteristics) and exposure to environmental factors (UV radiation, ionizing radiation) [6]. It seems that an individual genetic susceptibility has a greater impact on the development of multiple BCCs of the skin than the effect of extrinsic factors.

### 3.1 Genotypic characteristics

The principal genetic alterations mediating a predisposition to BCC development, especially multiple tumor manifestations, are not fully understood. DNA repair mechanisms play a critical role in protecting skin keratinocytes from UV mutagenesis and skin cancer development. Reduced DNA repair capacity was established as an independent risk factor for the development of BCC [7]. Except for UV, this defect can also be induced by genodermatoses (xeroderma pigmentosum), or germline defects in DNA repair genes [8] (i.e., XRCC3, APC, BARD1, BRCA1), especially among individuals who develop frequent, multiple BCCs [9]. Multiple BCC formation is also influenced by polymorphism of genes in a variety of molecular markers (e.g., cell-signaling proteins, carcinogen-metabolizing enzymes). In one study of BCC in the French population, BCC risk was associated with the PTCH c.3944C/C genotype, especially among patients with multiple BCCs [10]. MC1R is a key gene involved in pigmentation. Its variants constitute independent risk factors for the development of BCC with genetic dosage effect, through mechanisms of both pigmentation and non-pigmentation [10, 11]. Besides, MC1R variants have an influence on the number of BCC [12]. The same conclusion was drawn in another study among early-onset BCC [11]. A relationship has been demonstrated between glutathione S-transferase, cytochrome P450, reduced nicotinamide adenine dinucleotide NAD (+): quinone oxidoreductase, vitamin D receptor, tumor necrosis factor microsatellites, and the rate of a number of BCC lesions [13–16]. Polymorphisms in the genes encoding human leukocyte antigen (HLA) (e.g., HLA-DR4, HLA-DR1) are also implicated in the development of multiple BCC [17, 18].

Genetic syndromes, such as the Nevoid basal cell carcinoma, Bazex-Dupre-Christol syndrome, Rombo syndrome, xeroderma pigmentosum, and Bazex syndrome, are common inherited conditions with multiple, early onset BCC manifestations [19, 20]. Nevoid basal cell carcinoma (NBCCS), also known as Gorlin syndrome, is an autosomal dominant multisystem disorder with complete penetrance, and variable expression [21]. It is caused by mutations in the tumor suppressor genes patched (PTCH)1 gene, PTCH2 gene, and suppressor of the fused (SUFU) gene, and results in BCC in about 90% of those with the syndrome. Mutations in these genes, which are negative regulators of the Hedgehog (Hh) pathway, can lead to continuous activation of this pathway [22]. Additional mutated genes were found to be enriched in the major cilia components in NBCCS, such as IFT172 and KIFAP3, which encode ciliary proteins [23]. Since ciliary functions are fundamentally involved in the Hh signaling pathway, these gene alterations may be involved in the tumorigenesis of BCC. The UBE2A gene on the long arm of the X chromosome encodes a protein involved in repairing UV-damaged DNA and has been implicated in Bazex-Dupre-Christol syndrome [24]. The specific gene mutation associated with Rombo syndrome is still unknown. The phenotypes of Rombo syndrome and BDCS show a high degree of overlap [25]. Xeroderma pigmentosum is a group of conditions in which the nucleotide excision repair system is defective, so the body cannot adequately repair DNA damage from UV exposure. As a result, UV lesions are highly mutagenic and lead to skin cancers. Compared with the general population, patients with XP develop both BCC at higher frequencies [26]. Oculocutaneous albinism predisposes to malignant skin lesions, including BCC, due to pigmentary changes that render the individual highly susceptible to sun damage [27]. Brooke-Spiegler syndrome is an autosomal dominant disorder caused by CYLD gene mutations and characterized by multiple benign adnexal cutaneous neoplasms. Multiple nodular ulcerating BCCs in a patient with BSS were reported, inferring BCCs develop directly from trichoepitheliomas [28].

### 3.2 Phenotypic characteristics

In a cohort of 1239 BCCs from 728 single BCC and 171 multiple BCCs, male gender, tumor location in the trunk and upper extremities, and superficial histological subtype can be risk factors for a subsequent BCC [29]. And the male-to-female ratio continuously increased with the number of BCCs, consistent with previous research results [30, 31]. Other risk factors for developing multiple lesions in BCC include eye color, hair color, skin color, skin reaction with first summer sun exposure, and skin reaction with prolonged sun exposure [11]. Ethical differences also have been shown between single and multiple BCC. Tan ES et al. reported that Caucasians developed multiple BCC threefold more frequently than the Chinese in a prospective study [32]. An increased risk of new BCCs is seen in patients who already had a history of BCC [33]. Verkouteren JAC et al. developed a model to predict the absolute risk of a second BCC, based on the Fine and Gray regression model to account for the competing risk of death from other causes, indicating that having more than one initial BCC was the strongest predictor [34].

### 3.3 Ultraviolet radiation

UVR has been accepted as the key causal factor for cutaneous BCC, and a history of sunburn, especially grade II-III sunburns before adulthood was thought to be the major predisposing factor for multiple BCC, compared with single BCC [33]. Even indoor tanning was also associated with BCC, especially for multiple BCCs [35]. Depending on timing (childhood, adolescence), pattern (intermittent, continuous), source (natural, artificial), and amount (cumulative sun exposure), the impact of UVR on BCC development seems to be far more complex [36]. UV exposure is readily absorbed by DNA and induces the production of reactive oxygen species to damage DNA and trigger mutations in tumor suppressor genes, such as tp53 [37], TERT gene [38], and DPH3 gene [39]. UV exposure promotes inflammatory processes that encourage cancer growth, such as activation of NF-kB, toll-like receptors, Erbb2, and NLRP3 inflammasome; release of high-mobility group box-1; and enhancement of cyclooxygenase-2 expressions [40]. UVR can create a sustained immunosuppressive environment, one of the crucial parameters in the promotion and progression of photo-induced skin cancers, through antigen-presenting cell defect and altered cytokine environment in the draining lymph nodes [41]. Consistent evidence indicates that patients with a history of BCCs also have an elevated risk of developing other primary cutaneous malignancies [42].

### 3.4 Other environmental factors

Arsenic is a common cancer-causing chemical. The study conducted by Kibriya MG et al. suggested high arsenic exposure was associated with BCC through impaired DNA replication pathway, cellular response to DNA damage repair mechanism, and immune response at the genome-wide level [43].

### 3.5 Origin and clonality of multiple BCC

It is currently thought that the precursor cells for BCC originate from pluripotential stem cells in the basal layer of the interfollicular epidermis or the hair follicle [44]. But the question of the origin and clonality of multiple BCCs has not been clarified until now. Some studies suggested that the origin may be polyclonal and each BCC arises independently from a distinct progenitor cell. Heitzer et al. sequenced the PTCH gene and analyzed the LOH pattern of BCCs from a total of six patients with multiple lesions at different anatomical locations. They detected a total of 18 differential PTCH mutations in 14 of 18 BCCs [45]. While another molecular study of 41 BCC lesions from 15 female patients, assessing 9q LOH and X-chromosome inactivation patterns, contradicts such hypothesis and suggests that the majority of BCCs in an individual might originate from one single tumor cell clone [46].

### 3.6 Development of multiple BCC

In 2017, 46,226 patients were diagnosed with a first-ever primary BCC, and nearly one-quarter (n = 10,956) of these patients developed subsequent BCCs within the next 3 years (years 2017–2019) [47]. In a previous study, it was calculated that among individuals with at least 1 previous BCC, the 1-, 3-, and 5-year risk of a new BCC was 17%, 33%, and 41%, respectively [48].

The Hedgehog (Hh) pathway has an important role in the pathogenesis of BCC [49]. Most BCCs have been found to have mutations in different genes involved in the Hedgehog pathway, such as PTCH1, in Gorlin syndrome. This signaling pathway is crucial for the development of the embryo and fetus, involved in cell differentiation, cell growth, and morphogenesis. Hh signaling is also active in stem cells and tissues undergoing regeneration. It can be categorized as a canonical and noncanonical Hh pathway, considering whether a GLI-mediated transcription is involved. Sonic hedgehog is a ligand that binds to and inactivates the transmembrane PTCH, which normally inhibits Smoothened (SMO). When PTCH is inactivated by the binding of a sonic hedgehog, SMO is released and activates GLI proteins that serve as transcription factors in the nucleus for cell proliferation [50]. Recent research reveals that Hh signaling is also one of the crucial causes of the immunosuppressive tumor microenvironment, presenting as a lack of antitumor response pathways, downregulation of immune effectors, enrichment of immunosuppressive cells and chemokines, and activation of immunosuppressive signaling [51].

## 4. Clinical feature

Early basal cell carcinoma often appears as a single round or oval patch, indicating smoothness, and may be accompanied by scaling, telangiectasia, and pigmentation. A pearly papule with translucent margins typically characterizes it. Most BCCs grow slowly and are asymptomatic, often presenting as erosion or minor post-traumatic bleeding at first. Clinical features are diverse and include nodular, superficial, infiltrative, morpheaform (sclerosing), pigmented, and fibroepithelial types. The most common histological subtypes include nodular (nBCC), and superficial (sBCC) [52]. Nodular BCC accounts for about BCCs and 60–80% is most common in the head and neck. Nodular BCC appears as papules or nodules with telangiectasia. Superficial BCC accounts for about 20% of BCCs and is most common in the trunk and extremities. It is characterized by flat patches, often accompanied by scales, and partial atrophy. BCCs of the infiltrative type usually present clinically as a white-red patch with an unclear border and a hard texture, indicating an ulcerative scab. Morpheaform type BCC accounts for about 5–10% of BCCs. It occurs in the face and neck and often presents as an infiltrating plaque with unclear skin boundaries. BCC characterized by pigmentation is called pigmented Bcc, and all types can occur. Fibroepithelial type Bcc usually occurs in the back and is clinically manifested as skin-red papular nodules [53]. In addition, two syndromes are characterized by multiple BCC: nevoid basal cell carcinoma (NBCCS) and Bazex (Dupre-Christol) syndrome. NBCCS, also known as basal cell nevus syndrome (Gorlin syndrome), is a dominant genetic disease with frequent staining. Its clinical features include multiple BCC, keratocystic odontogenic tumors, hand-foot spot-like depression, and various skeletal and soft tissue abnormalities [54]. Qiu reported a case of a female patient who presented with multiple facial BCC-dominated NBCCS, which recovered well after surgical excision [55]. Bazex syndrome is characterized by numerous BCCs, follicular atrophoderma, congenital oligotrichosis, and local hypohidrosis [56]. Atilla [57] reported the case of a 70-year-old man suffering from Bazex (Dupre-Christol) syndrome. The patient presented with multiple BCC, accompanied by lung, pancreatic, and bladder cancer and hypohidrosis.

## 5. Diagnosis

### 5.1 Dermoscopic findings

Dermoscopy is a common noninvasive technique for the early diagnosis of BCC. It also allows for distinction between BCC subtypes and tumor management. The dermoscopic diagnosis of BCC is based on the presence of typical vascular structures, pigmented structures, and ulceration and the absence of specific melanocytic structures, including (a) branching and linear vessels (arborizing vessels/short fine telangiectasias), (b) blue-gray ovoid nests, (c) blue-gray globules and dots, (d) in-focus dots, (e) maple leaf-like areas, (f) spoke-wheel structures/areas, (g) concentric structures, (h) ulceration/ multiple small erosions, (i) absence of brown reticular lines (pigment network), (j) others: shiny white-red structureless areas and shiny white lines, circumferential stellate pattern, negative maple leaf-like structures, multiple aggregated yellow-white globules [58, 59]. The dermoscopic findings of multiple BCC, both syndromic and non-syndromic, on the same patient and in the same anatomical region were similar to those previously described in a single BCC [60–62].

Compared with single BCC, "white features" (i.e., white shiny lines, multiple yellow-white globules, and white circles and yellow clods) were less commonly observed in multiple BCC [33].

### 5.2 Histopathologic findings

Biopsy remains the gold standard for the diagnosis of BCCs. It only analyses high-risk BCCs or suspected lesions and requires invasive procedures. In general, BCC presents with blue islands, peripheral palisading, high nuclear/cytoplasmic ratio, retraction artifact, and fibro myxoid stroma. It can be subdivided into nonaggressive (superficial and nodular) and aggressive types (micronodular, infiltrative, morpheaform, and metatypical) in view of its histologic growth pattern. The ratio of nodular BCC was the largest in multiple BCC [29, 63, 64]. Compared with single BCC, the ratio of superficial BCC in multiple BCC was significantly higher. And there was a positive correlation between the nonaggressive histologic phenotype of BCC and multiple tumor presentation [8]. About 30% of GS cases have two or more types of BCC histopathological patterns (morphoea-like, solid, superficial, cystic, adenoid, fibroepithelial, pigmented) [65].

### 5.3 Reflectance confocal microscopy (RCM)

RCM is a noninvasive diagnostic technique that allows for *in vivo* visualization of the skin with a quasi-histological resolution of 0.5–1 μm, to a depth of about 150–200 μm. RCM has shown good sensitivity and specificity for the diagnosis of BCC, aiding in early diagnosis instead of biopsy [Diagnostic accuracy of confocal microscopy imaging vs. punch biopsy for diagnosing and subtyping basal cell carcinoma]. RCM has revealed that the BCC tumor islands have areas of low refractility, presenting as multiple, small islands of basaloid cells with multilobular architecture. Peripheral palisading of nuclei, highly refractile fibrous tissue (superficial dermis, bright inflammatory cells, telangiectasia), and peritumoral dark spaces can also be found [66].

Manubens E et al. performed a complete and sensitive diagnosis of a multiple BCC patient with 26 lesions using RCM that were equivocal with dermoscopy in only 29 and 33 min at pre- and posttreatment, respectively [67]. RCM's main limitation is the inability to image at deeper layers of the dermis.

### 5.4 Optical coherence tomography (OCT)

OCT evolves as an effective noninvasive imaging modality used to diagnose and evaluate BCCs, which generates cross-sectional images. While it lacks cellular resolution, it can image at depths of 1000–2000 μm, comparable to biopsy. Under OCT, BCCs were visualized as hypoechoic structures but showed a mixed echogenicity, some with peripheral rimming and disruption of the epidermis [68]. The total time taken to scan all 24 lesions of a Gorlin syndrome patient was under 30 min through OCT [69]. Compared with traditional OCT images, line-field confocal optical coherence tomography produced a higher agreement (90.4%) of the BCC subtype and conventional histology, which allows for a cellular resolution (axial 1.1"m, lateral 1.2"m) and a depth up to the mid-dermis (approximately 500"m) in its images [70]. A handheld single-fiber OCT instrument can precisely correlate OCT findings and anatomic locations, allowing the surgeon to achieve a negative margin more confidently after 1 excision stage in Mohs micrographic surgery [71].

### 5.5 Ultrasonography

Ultrasound's accessibility, noninvasive nature, safety, and ability to provide information in real-time make it an invaluable tool in the assessment of BCCs. The operator can manage the detection depth through variable frequency probes of the technique. Performance of high-frequency ultrasound (HFUS, e.g., ≥15 MHz) or ultra-high frequency ultrasound (UHFUS, e.g., 30 MHz up to 100 MHz) with high definition and penetration that generates well-demarcated images [72]. Ultrasound's Morphological Characteristics of BCCs include Surface Measurements, Depth, Margins, and Invasion [73]. BCCs appear on ultrasound as a hypoechoic dermal or subdermal structure of variable shape that often contains tumoral hyperechoic spots. Hyperechoic spots were very informative to stratify BCCs by severity and to identify certain specific subtypes [74].

### 5.6 Others

Recently, RCM and OCT have been combined to test for the diagnosis of BCC in a prospective study. In this study with 32 single BCC and 3 multiple BCCs, RCM-OCT showed an overall agreement of 91.1% with Mohs micrographic surgery-frozen sections, a sensitivity of 82.6%, specificity of 93.8% for the diagnosis of residual BCC and margin evaluation [75]. RCM-OCT takes advantage of the higher cellular resolution of RCM and the ability to measure up to 1000 μm with OCT, which helps in the evaluation of BCCs [76].

## 6. Pretreatment assessment

Assessing the risk level of the lesion is the most important step in the choice of treatment modality for basal cell carcinoma and should avoid the serious consequences of overtreatment or inadequate treatment. Because basal cell carcinoma is often confined to the local area, TNM staging is not often used. Basal cell carcinoma is classified as high-risk or low-risk based on lesion site and lesion size, border, primary or recurrent, presence or absence of immunosuppression, whether it is a site of prior radiation therapy, type of pathology, and presence or absence of perineural infiltration. The more high-risk factors a patient contains, the higher the risk level and the worse the prognosis. Multiple basal cell carcinomas are mainly caused by excessive exposure of the skin to UV radiation. Physical examination should carefully examine the head, face, neck, arms, and back of the hands. We reported a 54-year-old male patient with multiple BCCs of the perioral region who had a history of pulmonary nodule surgery (**Figure 1**). Images were captured by VISIA facial imaging booth (VISIA-CR, Canfield). In physical examination, nodules with pearly-like surfaces and arborizing vessels were observed above the left lip, below the left lip, below the right lip, and in the middle of the lower lip; there presented ivory-white, smooth, and scar-like depressions above the right lip; the nodules in the middle of the lower lip and the depressions above the right lip extended past the vermilion border into the lip; other skin regions were not involved. This patient was exempted from nevoid basal cell carcinoma syndrome (NBCCS) and did not have a history of radiotherapy. The diagnosis of multiple BCCs was finally confirmed through skin biopsy at multiple sites. This patient did not have NBCCS or receive radiotherapy before. Multiple BCCs distributed around the perioral region seem to be related to shaving. Multiple BCCs may be associated with male gender, age, nodular BCCs, or facial involvement at the time of the first diagnosis,

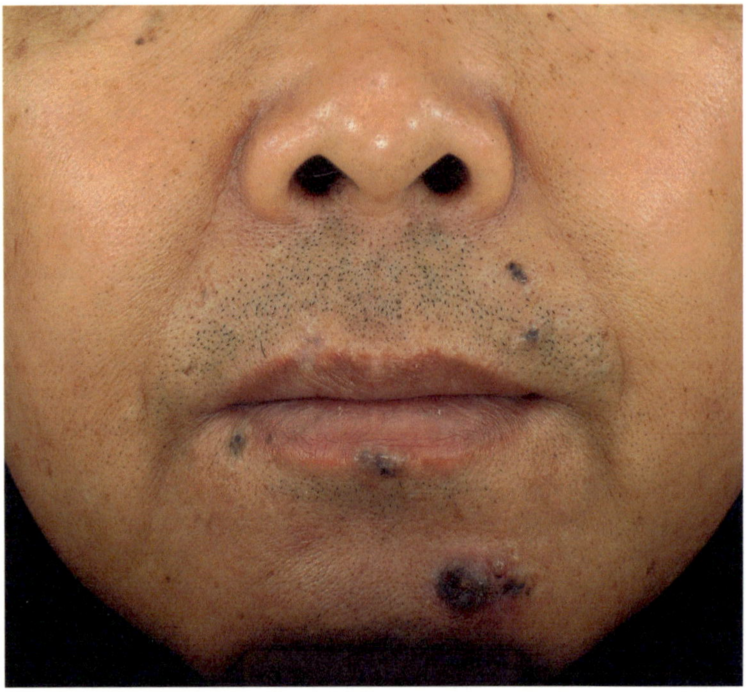

**Figure 1.**
*A case of 54-year-old male patient with multiple BCCs of the perioral region.*

according to the multivariate analysis [64]. A positive family history of skin cancer is an important factor in the development of basal cell carcinoma. Appropriate evaluation for genetic disorders should also be performed. Germline mutations in the PTCH1 gene are present in patients with Gorlin syndrome or basal cell carcinoma naevus syndrome. The Gorlin syndrome is an autosomal dominant disorder characterized by skeletal abnormalities, jaw cysts, and multiple basal cell carcinoma of the skin. An inherited mutation in the tumor suppressor gene causes multiple basal cell carcinomas in conjunction with Gorlin syndrome [77]. In order to prevent life-long complications of this syndrome, early diagnosis is crucial to counseling patients, including malignancy, oro-maxillofacial deformation, and destruction. This can be reduced by diagnosing and treating at the earliest possible time [78]. There is a higher prevalence in kidney transplant patients than in the general population. More than half of solid organ transplant recipients will develop nonmelanoma skin cancer, such as basal cell carcinoma or squamous cell carcinoma, at some point in their lives [79]. Based on nonlinear image analysis techniques, the study observed differences that underscore the relevance of T-cell suppression in cancer behavior [80]. Immunosuppression is a significant risk factor [81]. Basal cell carcinoma is the second most common skin cancer in posttransplant patients [82]. A review of the history of medically-derived immunosuppressive drug use is equally important. Because basal cell carcinoma includes a large number of subtypes, it is also important to differentiate between the manifestations of the various subtypes. The study examined the relationship between multiple basal cell carcinomas and internal malignant neoplasms among 199 patients with multiple basal cell carcinoma presented with no substantial deviations [83]. The factors are complex and still not completely understood. Multiple basal cell carcinomas arising from epidermal nevus also need to evaluate [84].

## 7. Therapy

### 7.1 Surgical treatment

Surgical treatment is the standard of care for most BCCs. Standard surgical excision is suitable for low-risk BCC, and for lesions <20 mm in diameter, a 4 mm surgical margin is recommended, with a low risk of recurrence after standard excision. Mohs micrographic surgery allows for maximum preservation of normal tissue to meet functional and esthetic needs but is more costly and not suitable for low-risk BCC. Complete circumferential peripheral and deep margin assessment is also suitable for high-risk BCC. However, the surgical treatment of multiple basal cell carcinomas is still not sufficiently studied, especially for Gorlin syndrome or basal cell carcinoma naevus syndrome. The cases of multiple sporadic, nonsyndromic BCCs were reported completely removed by surgery [85]. A re-excision with wider margins is recommended if incompletely excised lesions recur, as the risk of multiple recurrences is as high as 50%. Following surgical excision, reconstruction should be the primary consideration in cases of multiple defects. In general, full-thickness skin grafts and flaps can be used for repair. We reported a design using an equal area splicing for the reconstruction of multiple defects after the excision of multiple basal cell carcinomas [86]. The donor site was designed according to the size and shape of the skin defect. In the donor site, the double semicircle dislocation splicing method was used as the first level design, and then the second level design within the double semicircular skin graft was carried out according to the area measurement and morphological evaluation of the skin graft defect. In exceptional cases, if one-stage repair is not possible, treatment can be performed by second-stage healing. The healing pattern of multiple basal cell carcinoma should depend on the size, depth, and location of the defects.

### 7.2 Curettage and electrodesiccation

Curettage and electrodesiccation (C&ED) is the process of removing tumor tissue with a curettage device and denaturing the tissue by electrodesiccation C&ED. This method is simple in clinical operation, has a low economic burden for patients, and is suitable for low-risk BCCs [87]. The cure rate of C&ED can reach 91–97% if suitable lesions are selected after 5 years of follow-up. However, many studies have shown that C&ED may have a high recurrence rate (19–27%). It may be attributed to the selection of high-risk areas and tissue subtype correlation [53]. Since this procedure does not assess histopathological margins, it is not recommended in areas with terminal hair growth, such as the scalp, beard, and pubic bone [3]. Tumors deep below the hair follicle structure may fail to be removed using C&ED. If the cancer is found to have developed into the subcutaneous layer, C&ED should not be used and surgery is most appropriate. And in low-risk tumor areas, it is advisable to send the curettage to biopsy to guide subsequent treatment [88]. This procedure tests the doctor's skill level and is prone to scarring. It should be avoided on the face. Fournier et al. [89] showed that the curettage-electrodesiccation group was better than the curettage cryosurgery group in the treatment of basal cell carcinoma or squamous cell carcinoma, and the recurrence rate was lower.

### 7.3 5-fluorouracil

By inhibiting enzymes, 5-fluorouracil can affect DNA synthesis and achieve the purpose of antitumor. Topical 5-fluorouracil is easy to operate, inexpensive, and effective. It is the first topical drug approved for the treatment of superficial BCCs [90]. 5-fluorouracil creams are available in 5, 10, and 20% concentrations, with 5% recommended for superficial BCCs. Topical 5-fluorouracil cream is recommended twice a day for 3–6 weeks [91]. Gross et al. [90] used 5% 5-fluorouracil cream to treat 31 patients with superficial BCC and achieved a 90% cure rate with few adverse reactions and high patient satisfaction. Studies in Diluviol [92] have shown that 5% 5-fluorouracil cream combined with 10% salicylic acid can effectively treat pigmentary BCC, but no large sample studies are required. Naik et al. [93] used topical 5-fluorouracil cream to treat facial multiple basal cell carcinoma and achieved a good effect, with no recurrence after 6 months of follow-up. Studies have shown that topical 5-fluorouracil is suitable for recurrent BCCs with lesions more significant than 10 mm in diameter and borderless clearness. However, it should be noted that 5-fluorouracil should not be used around the eyelids due to its corneal toxicity. In addition, Avant et al. [94] showed that intradermal injection of 5-fluorouracil was effective in treating invasive BCC. The usual dose is 1–3 ml for injection, and the endpoint reaction is the whiteness of the lesion. Before injection, 0.5 ml of 1% lidocaine is injected locally.

### 7.4 Imiquimod

Imiquimod is a synthetic agent that stimulates the production of cytokines, including interferon, by activating toll-like receptors (TLR)-7 on antigen-presenting cells for antiproliferative and antitumor effects. Topical imiquimod 5% cream is suitable for the treatment of sBCC, and the recommended course of treatment is once a day, 5 days a week for 6 weeks [95]. Ruiz et al. [96] applied 5% imiquimod cream three times a week for 4 weeks in 82 patients with sBCC and achieved an 85% clearance rate after 2 years of follow-up. A randomized, controlled, multicenter study of 99 cases of sBCCs treated with topical 5% imiquimod cream achieved good results after 6 weeks. The results showed a twice-daily clearance rate of 100%, and only one patient dropped out of the study due to adverse skin reactions [97]. Jansen [98] randomly divided sBcc patients into topical imiquimod cream, fluorouracil, and photodynamic therapy (MAL-PDT) groups. In this study, 601 patients with sBCC were followed up for 5 years. The results showed that topical imiquimod cream was superior to fluorouracil and MAL-PDT. A study of 17 BCC patients with manifestations of Gorlins syndrome treated with 5% imiquimod cream achieved a 77% cure rate with no recurrence [99]. One patient with multiple superficial BCC did not respond to 5% fluorouracil cream, while topical imiquimod cream locally subsided [100]. A study of 67 patients with multiple superficial BCCs showed a 77% cure rate with topical imiquimod 5% cream. The study also found that the clearance rate of lower limbs was the worst compared with other sites, suggesting there may be a heterogeneity of treatment sites [101].

### 7.5 Intralesional injection

Intralesional injection enables drugs to act on the lesion directly, penetrate deeper, and avoid systemic toxicity and surgical complications. The intralesional injection is usually used for patients who are not candidates for surgery, especially with high recurrence risk. Several agents for BCC intralesional injection therapy have been studied with a high degree of efficacy, including 5-fluorouracil, interferon, interleukin-2, and bleomycin, but the evidence of long-term efficacy is limited. For example, 5-fluorouracil is a pyrimidine analog whose cytotoxic metabolites are incorporated into DNA and RNA, inducing cell cycle arrest and apoptosis. It has been widely used in malignant tumors, but there is no clinical trial data on the treatment of multiple basal cell carcinoma. Only a case reported a 62-year-old male patient from China who was diagnosed with multiple basal cell carcinoma by skin biopsy and genetic testing. He finally chose 5-FU (0.25 g/10 ml) intralesional injection combined with 30% salicylic acid and 5% 5-FU ointment for external use after local lesion curettage because of the high incidence of head and face and economic burden. No recurrence was observed under follow-up until half a year later [102]. Bleomycin, an antibiotic produced by Streptomyces verticillate, causes the scission of DNA and inhibition of DNA ligase. A clinical study of electrochemical therapy using bleomycin combined with an electric pulse in the treatment of multiple basal cell carcinoma, including a total of 54 lesions with an average diameter of 0.91 cm (range 0.37 ~ 2.1 cm) from 20 patients. Intralesional injection with bleomycin (tumor volume below 100 $mm^3$ injected 0.5-unit bleomycin; 0.75 unit between 100 and 150 $mm^3$, and 1.0 unit above 150 $mm^3$), followed by electrical pulse therapy. The final complete remission rate was as high as 98, 94% of lesions achieved complete remission after a single treatment, and no recurrence was observed after an 18-month follow-up [103]. An 82-year-old woman presented with multiple lesions in the right temporal region that were not responsive to radiotherapy. Bleomycin was injected into eight new histopathological confirmed basal cell carcinoma lesions, and 7 intralesional injections of 3 IU bleomycin were administered every 48 hours. No recurrence or new lesions were observed in the follow-up within 2 years [104]. However, the evidence for the treatment of multiple cell carcinoma by intralesional injection is still limited, and its effectiveness still needs more randomized controlled clinical studies to verify.

### 7.6 Cryotherapy

Cryotherapy uses the physical properties of the refrigerant substance, the low temperature acts on the lesions to achieve the removal of malignant tissue. It was first used as the treatment of basal cell carcinoma as early as the nineteenth century [105]. It's the first choice for patients who want to avoid invasive surgery and is suitable for the treatment of low-risk multiple basal cell carcinoma. However, it's not recommended for patients with lesions below the knee. Some clinicians recommend using curettage, and electrodesiccation to reduce the tumor volume before cryotherapy, or combined with other methods when the efficacy is under expectations. In a case report, a 58-year-old man with superficial multiple basal cell carcinoma with different sizes in the chest, back, and waist, cryotherapy alone or combined with 5-fluorouracil was tried, and no recurrence was found after 6 months of follow-up [106]. The curative effectiveness of cryotherapy has a great discrepancy in different published studies [107–110]. A prospective clinical randomized controlled trial studied the effectiveness of cryotherapy in superficial multiple basal cell carcinoma, and the results showed that the clinical clearance rate of cryotherapy was as high as 100% after 1 year ($P = 0.060$) [111]. There are also systematic reviews reported that the efficacy and safety of cryotherapy alone or cryotherapy combined with curettage in the treatment of primary superficial basal cell carcinoma and nodular basal cell carcinoma are comparable to photodynamic therapy, but the postoperative esthetics of patients is not as good as photodynamic therapy [112]. Of course, cryotherapy has some limitations, besides common side effects, such as erythema, blisters, and pain, there are also many other complications such as hypertrophic scars and postinflammatory pigment changes. Notably, recurrent cancer lesions may be covered by fibrous scar tissue, resulting in extensive tumor infiltration.

### 7.7 Photodynamic therapy

Photodynamic therapy (PDT) and oral vismodegib provide noninvasive treatments for basal cell carcinomas (BCCs) in widespread BCCs and patients who are poor surgical candidates. Different types of BCC respond differently to PDT, with superficial BCC being the most sensitive to treatment. Combining PDT with vismodegib may be a safe and effective therapy for the treatment of multiple BCCs [113]. A genetic mutation in PTCH1 c.1804C > T (p.Arg602*) results in Chinese nevoid basal cell carcinoma syndrome associated with multiple basal cell carcinoma phenotypes. Multiple modalities, including microwave ablation, photodynamic therapy, and excision surgery, have a good response to the nevoid basal cell carcinoma syndrome [114]. A case of numerous nodular BCCs scattered on the face and head was treated with topical curettage and modified ALA-PDT. Curettage was to rapidly scalp away nodular tumors and contributed to ALA transdermal depth to the tumor base [115]. We also reported a case of multiple basal cell carcinomas scattered on the leg, with successful treatment with surgical excision, topical curettage, and modified ALA-PDT (**Figure 2A-D**). The combination of surgery and photodynamic therapy is a safe and effective treatment for multiple basal cell carcinomas [116]. Patients with multiple superficial lesions may benefit from PDT.

### 7.8 Laser therapy

Ablative lasers are effective in treating superficial, low-risk BCC, with the advantages of less pain, faster recovery, convenient operation, and better cosmetic effect. For example, the CO2 laser can be used to treat multiple basal cell carcinomas of 2–4 mm in children [117], with endpoints of dermal tightening and slight crust formation, without bleeding or tissue reaction outside the treated area. Related studies have shown that abnormal expression of chemokines correlates significantly with angiogenesis in the tumor mesenchyme [118]. And the theory of selective photothermal action supports the possibility of using vascular-selective laser destruction of blood vessels to treat multiple basal cell carcinomas [119]. For example, it

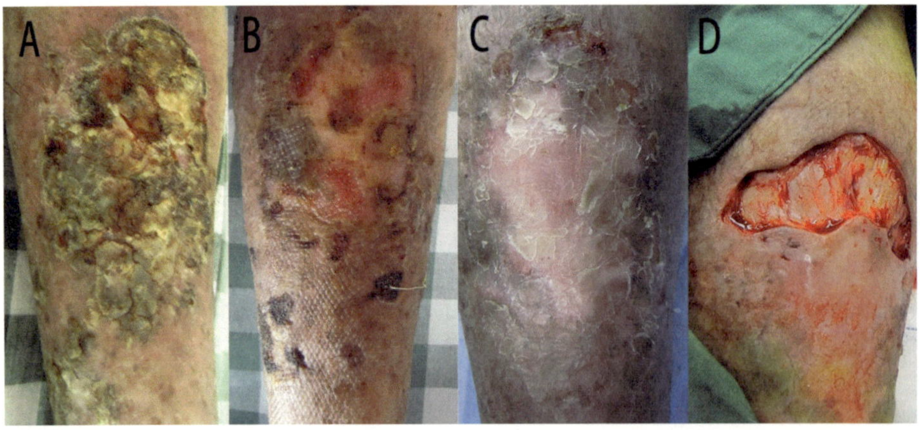


**Figure 2.**
*A case of successful treatment with multiple basal cell carcinomas. A. multiple basal cell carcinomas scattered on the leg, B-C. Modified ALA-PDT with topical curettage, D. the areas of resistant to modified ALA-PDT are treated surgically for eradication.*

has been reported that a single treatment with the long-pulsed 755 nm alexandrite laser can achieve both clinical and histopathological clearance of multiple basal cell carcinoma lesions. The wavelength 595 nm PDL selectively destroys dermal blood vessels of 0.75 ~ 1.25 mm thickness by photothermal action, and the clinical efficiency can range from 62 to 95% [120–122]. On account of only a few cases of various types of lasers have been reported for the treatment of multiple basal cell carcinoma, and there are no randomized controlled trials to prove the effectiveness of these methods, we are unable to accurately assess Laser therapy efficiency in the treatment of multiple basal cell carcinoma.

### 7.9 Radiotherapy

Radiotherapy can be used as a complementary therapy for aggressive or high-risk BCC that is not amenable to surgery, especially in those with perineural involvement. Radiotherapy has the advantage of avoiding invasive procedures and is indicated for patients for whom surgery is contraindicated or who are without a strong desire for surgery. However, radiotherapy is mostly not recommended in multiple basal cell carcinoma and is even contraindicated in conventional treatment. Because of its inability to control the edge, poor cosmetic outcomes, and long treatment period. Also, many studies suggest that long-term radiotherapy increases the high risk of developing skin cancer [123–125]. However, several studies have reported that patients with Gorlin syndrome had no signs of recurrence at an average follow-up of 6 months after radiation therapy, and no cases of secondary skin malignancies after radiation therapy were observed [126, 127]. Related studies have shown that the relative risk of developing BCC after radiation therapy in children is higher, and the susceptibility to secondary malignancies is similarly higher in children with Gorlin syndrome than in adults [128, 129], so radiotherapy is generally chosen for patients over 60 years of age.

### 7.10 Itraconazole

Itraconazole is an agent that binds SMO protein to inhibit the Hh pathway. In addition, itraconazole stops the cell cycle, inhibits angiogenesis, and leads to apoptosis and autophagy [130]. The side effects are commonly related to the gastrointestinal tract [131]. Kim DJ et al. observed 57 primary BCCs in eight patients were down 24% [132]. As is reported, Itraconazole and arsenic trioxide, alone or combined, inhibit the growth of medulloblastoma and basal cell carcinoma *in vivo* and prolong the survival of mice suffering from intracranial drug-resistant SMO D477G medulloblastoma [133]. In an exploratory phase II trial of oral itraconazole for the treatment of multiple BCCs, itraconazole reduced cell proliferation by 45%, HH pathway activity by 65%, and tumor zone by 24% [134].

### 7.11 Targeted therapy

The Hedgehog pathway plays a vital role in multiple BCCs. This pathway is largely maintained with the exception of hair follicles, skin, and stem cells, which is essential for proliferation, differentiation, and maintenance [135]. On the one hand, this pathway goes through a paracrine mechanism to support tumor growth. On the other hand, the activation of Hh signaling in surrounding fibroblasts promotes the mobilization of neoplastic stroma by tumor cells [136]. Recently, FDA has approved vismodegib, sonidegib, and patidegib, three Hedgehog pathway inhibitors, to treat patients with advanced BCCs. These drugs inhibit smoothened, a hyperactive transmembrane protein by a homologous protein, which plays a key role in Hh signal transduction [136]. PTCH1 secrets PTCH protein and inhibits SMO signaling [137]. Therefore, no signals reach the nucleus to inhibit the Hh pathway. As was reported, vismodegib and sonidegib displayed a total response rate of up to approximately 70% and still >50% in the locally advanced context, and adverse events have been reported for muscular spasms, alopecia, and dysgeusia [138]. Dennis Niebel et al. reported a case of a 67-year-old female with multiple BCCs of the scalp who had a fascinating partial remission after 3 months with vismodegib and sonidegib [139]. Abnormal activation of the Hedgehog pathway is a molecular driver of basal cell carcinoma, with most bccs carrying somatic point mutations, mainly UV-induced heterozygosity and/or copy loss of the PTCH1 gene. Recently, mutation and function analysis showed that PTPN14 and LATS1 and MYCN were new BCC-associated genes. In addition, emerging reports have found frequent noncoding mutations in the regulatory promoter sequences of the TERT and DPH3-OXNAD1 genes. Therefore, new molecular-targeted therapies are still being studied [2].

## 8. Conclusion

Despite progress in recent years, treating multiple basal cell carcinomas still remains challenging and there is plenty of room for a systemic approach. Further studies will improve our knowledge about this disease and the therapeutic options available to treat it. The understanding of molecular events implicated in their development has allowed the development of new strategies.

## Acknowledgements

First of all, I would like to give my heartfelt thanks to all the people who have ever helped me with this paper. I am also extremely grateful to all my friends and classmates who have kindly provided me with assistance and companionship in the course of preparing this paper. Finally, I am really grateful to all those who devote much time to reading this thesis and give me much advice, which will benefit me in my later study.

## Conflict of interest

The authors declare no conflict of interest.

**Author details**

Qiaochu Zhou*, Yanan Zhang, Shan Zhang, Jinhui Wang, Lele Lin and Jie Xu
Wenzhou Hospital of Integrated Traditional Chinese and Western Medicine, Affiliated Hospital of Integrated Traditional Chinese and Western Medicine of Shanghai University, Wenzhou, China

*Address all correspondence to: transferzhou@sina.com

## References

[1] Basset-Seguin N, Herms F. Update in the management of basal cell carcinoma. Acta Dermato-Venereologica. 2020;**100**(11):adv00140

[2] Pellegrini C, Maturo MG, Di Nardo L, Ciciarelli V, Gutiérrez García-Rodrigo C, Fargnoli MC. Understanding the molecular genetics of basal cell carcinoma. International Journal of Molecular Sciences. 2017;**18**(11):2485 Published 2017 Nov 22

[3] Paoli J, Gyllencreutz JD, Fougelberg J, et al. Nonsurgical options for the treatment of basal cell carcinoma. Dermatology Practical & Conceptual. 2019;**9**(2):75-81

[4] Ozkanli S, Soylemez T, Keskin H, et al. A five-year retrospective analysis of basal cell carcinoma: A monocentric study. Medeniyet Medical Journal. 2020;**35**(3):219-225

[5] Soutou B, Massih C, Sleilaty G, et al. Clinical and pathological features associated with high-risk, multiple, and recurrent basal cell carcinomas: A retrospective cohort analysis from the Levantine coast of the Mediterranean Sea. Archives of Dermatological Research. 2023;**315**(1):51-59

[6] Ligeralde-Bascones KI, Gulmatico-Flores Z, Lim-Bueser HG, et al. Diagnosis and management of basal cell carcinoma: Interdisciplinary consensus statements of Jose R. Reyes memorial medical Center, a Department of Health Tertiary Hospital in Manila, Philippines. International Journal of Dermatology. 2022;**10**.1111/ijd.16555

[7] Wang LE, Li C, Strom SS, et al. Repair capacity for UV light induced DNA damage associated with risk of nonmelanoma skin cancer and tumor progression. Clinical Cancer Research. 2007;**13**:6532-6539

[8] Köberle B, Koch B, Fischer BM, et al. Single nucleotide polymorphisms in DNA repair genes and putative cancer risk. Archives of Toxicology. 2016;**90**(10):2369-2388

[9] Cho HG, Kuo KY, Li S, et al. Frequent basal cell cancer development is a clinical marker for inherited cancer susceptibility. JCI Insight. 2018;**3**(15):e122744

[10] Liboutet M, Portela M, Delestaing G, et al. MC1R and PTCH gene polymorphism in French patients with basal cell carcinomas. The Journal of Investigative Dermatology. 2006;**126**(7):1510-1517

[11] Ferrucci LM, Cartmel B, Molinaro AM, et al. Host phenotype characteristics and MC1R in relation to early-onset basal cell carcinoma. The Journal of Investigative Dermatology. 2012;**132**(4):1272-1279

[12] Bastiaens MT, ter Huurne JA, Kielich C, et al. Leiden skin cancer study team. Melanocortin-1 receptor gene variants determine the risk of nonmelanoma skin cancer independently of fair skin and red hair. American Journal of Human Genetics. 2001;**68**(4):884-894

[13] Lear JT, Heagerty AH, Smith A, et al. Multiple cutaneous basal cell carcinomas: Glutathione S-transferase (GSTM1, GSTT1) and cytochrome P450 (CYP2D6, CYP1A1) polymorphisms influence tumour numbers and accrual. Carcinogenesis. 1996;**17**(9):1891-1896

[14] Clairmont A, Sies H, Ramachandran S, et al. Association of NAD(P)H:Quinone

oxidoreductase (NQO1) null with numbers of basal cell carcinomas: Use of a multivariate model to rank the relative importance of this polymorphism and those at other relevant loci. Carcinogenesis. 1999;**20**:1235-1240

[15] Hajeer AH, Lear JT, Ollier WE, et al. Preliminary evidence of an association of tumour necrosis factor microsatellites with increased risk of multiple basal cell carcinomas. The British Journal of Dermatology. 2000;**142**(3):441-445

[16] Ramachandran S, Fryer AA, Lovatt TJ, et al. Combined effects of gender, skin type and polymorphic genes on clinical phenotype: Use of rate of increase in numbers of basal cell carcinomas as a model system. Cancer Letters. 2003;**189**:175-181

[17] Czarnecki D, Nicholson I, Tait B, et al. HLA DR4 is associated with the development of multiple basal cell carcinomas and malignant melanoma. Dermatology. 1993;**187**:16-18

[18] Czarnecki D, Lewis A, Nicholson I, et al. Multiple basal cell carcinomas and HLA frequencies in southern Australia. Journal of the American Academy of Dermatology. 1991;**24**:559-561

[19] Schierbeck J, Vestergaard T, Bygum A. Skin cancer associated genodermatoses: A literature review. Acta Dermato-Venereologica. 2019;**99**(4):360-369

[20] Parren LJ, Frank J. Hereditary tumour syndromes featuring basal cell carcinomas. The British Journal of Dermatology. 2011;**165**(1):30-34

[21] Kimonis VE, Goldstein AM, Pastakia B, et al. Clinical manifestations in 105 persons with nevoid basal cell carcinoma syndrome. American Journal of Medical Genetics. 1997;**69**(3):299-308

[22] Durmaz CD, Evans G, Smith MJ, et al. A novel PTCH1 frameshift mutation leading to nevoid basal cell carcinoma syndrome. Cytogenetic and Genome Research. 2018;**154**:57-61

[23] Onodera S, Morita N, Nakamura Y, et al. Novel alterations in IFT172 and KIFAP3 may induce basal cell carcinoma. Orphanet Journal of Rare Diseases. 2021;**16**(1):443

[24] AlSabbagh MM, Baqi MA. Bazex-Dupré-Christol syndrome: Review of clinical and molecular aspects. International Journal of Dermatology. 2018;**57**(9):1102-1106

[25] van Steensel MA, Jaspers NG, Steijlen PM. A case of Rombo syndrome. The British Journal of Dermatology. 2001;**144**(6):1215-1218

[26] Dupuy A, Sarasin A. DNA damage and gene therapy of xeroderma pigmentosum, a human DNA repair-deficient disease. Mutation Research. 2015;**776**:2-8

[27] Hassan S, Louis SJ, Fethiere M, et al. The prevalence of nonmelanoma skin cancer in a population of patients with oculocutaneous albinism in Haiti. International Journal of Dermatology. 2022;**61**(7):867-871

[28] Shiver M, Hughes M, Naylor M, et al. A novel CYLD gene mutation and multiple basal cell carcinomas in a patient with Brooke-Spiegler syndrome. Clinical and Experimental Dermatology. 2016;**41**(1):98-100

[29] Bartos V, Kullova M. Basal cell carcinoma multiplicity - a retrospective analysis of 899 biopsy-proven patients from a single institute. Klinická Onkologie. 2017;**30**(3):197-201

[30] Flohil SC, Koljenović S, de Haas ER, et al. Cumulative risks and rates of

subsequent basal cell carcinomas in the Netherlands. The British Journal of Dermatology. 2011;**165**(4):874-881

[31] Souza CF, Thomé EP, Menegotto PF, et al. Topography of basal cell carcinoma and their correlations with gender, age and histologic pattern: A retrospective study of 1042 lesions. Anais Brasileiros de Dermatologia. 2011;**86**(2):272-277

[32] Tan ES, Ee M, Shen L, et al. Basal cell carcinoma in Singapore: A prospective study on epidemiology and clinicopathological characteristics with a secondary comparative analysis between Singaporean Chinese and Caucasian patients. The Australasian Journal of Dermatology. 2015;**56**(3):175-179

[33] Sgouros D, Rigopoulos D, Panayiotides I, et al. Novel insights for patients with multiple basal cell carcinomas and tumors at high-risk for recurrence: Risk factors, clinical morphology, and dermatoscopy. Cancers (Basel). 2021;**13**(13):3208

[34] Verkouteren JAC, Smedinga H, Steyerberg EW, et al. Predicting the risk of a second basal cell carcinoma. The Journal of Investigative Dermatology. 2015;**135**(11):2649-2656

[35] Ferrucci LM, Cartmel B, Molinaro AM, et al. Indoor tanning and risk of early-onset basal cell carcinoma. Journal of the American Academy of Dermatology. 2012;**67**(4):552-562

[36] Göppner D, Leverkus M. Basal cell carcinoma: From the molecular understanding of the pathogenesis to targeted therapy of progressive disease. Journal of Skin Cancer. 2011;**2011**:650258

[37] Kumar R, Deep G, Agarwal R. An overview of ultraviolet B radiation-induced skin cancer chemoprevention by silibinin. Current Pharmacology Reports. 2015;**1**(3):206-215

[38] Pópulo H, Boaventura P, Vinagre J, et al. TERT promoter mutations in skin cancer: The effects of sun exposure and X-irradiation. The Journal of Investigative Dermatology. 2014;**134**(8):2251-2257

[39] Denisova E, Heidenreich B, Nagore E, et al. Frequent DPH3 promoter mutations in skin cancers. Oncotarget. 2015;**6**(34):35922-35930

[40] Teng Y, Yu Y, Li S, et al. Ultraviolet radiation and basal cell carcinoma: An environmental perspective. Frontiers in Public Health. 2021;**9**:666528

[41] Hart PH, Grimbaldeston MA, Finlay-Jones JJ. Sunlight, immunosuppression and skin cancer: Role of histamine and mast cells. Clinical and Experimental Pharmacology & Physiology. 2001;**28**(1-2):1-8

[42] Flohil SC, van der Leest RJ, Arends LR, et al. Risk of subsequent cutaneous malignancy in patients with prior keratinocyte carcinoma: A systematic review and meta-analysis. European Journal of Cancer. 2013;**49**:2365-2375

[43] Kibriya MG, Jasmine F, Munoz A, et al. Interaction of arsenic exposure and transcriptomic profile in basal cell carcinoma. Cancers (Basel). 2022;**14**(22):5598

[44] Sehgal VN, Chatterjee K, Pandhi D, et al. Basal cell carcinoma: Pathophysiology. Skinmed. 2014;**12**:176-181

[45] Heitzer E, Quehenberger F, Wolf P. Polyclonality of multiple sporadic basal cell carcinomas. The Journal of Investigative Dermatology. 2009;**129**:1586-1589

[46] Shulman O, Laitman Y, Vilan A, et al. Monoclonal origin of anatomically

distinct basal cell carcinomas. The Journal of Investigative Dermatology. 2006;**126**:676-679

[47] Schreuder K, Hollestein L, Nijsten TEC, et al. A nationwide study of the incidence and trends of first and multiple basal cell carcinomas in the Netherlands and prediction of future incidence. The British Journal of Dermatology. 2022;**186**(3):476-484

[48] Karagas MR, Stukel TA, Greenberg ER, et al. Risk of subsequent basal cell carcinoma and squamous cell carcinoma of the skin among patients with prior skin cancer. Skin cancer prevention study group. JAMA. 1992;**267**:3305-3310

[49] Tampa M, Georgescu SR, Mitran CI, et al. Recent advances in signaling pathways comprehension as carcinogenesis triggers in basal cell carcinoma. Journal of Clinical Medicine. 2020;**9**(9):3010

[50] Pietrobono S, Gagliardi S, Stecca B. Non-canonical hedgehog signaling pathway in cancer: Activation of GLI transcription factors beyond smoothened. Frontiers in Genetics. 2019;**10**:556

[51] Jiang J, Ding Y, Chen Y, et al. Pan-cancer analyses reveal that increased hedgehog activity correlates with tumor immunosuppression and resistance to immune checkpoint inhibitors. Cancer Medicine. 2022;**11**(3):847-863

[52] Telfer NR, Colver GB, Morton CA. Guidelines for the management of basal cell carcinoma. British Journal of Dermatology. 2010;**159**(1):35-48

[53] Naik PP, Desai MB. Basal cell carcinoma: A narrative review on contemporary diagnosis and management. Oncology and Therapy. 2022;**10**(2):317-335

[54] Bresler SC, Padwa BL, Granter SR. Nevoid basal cell carcinoma syndrome (Gorlin syndrome). Head and Neck Pathology. 2016;**10**(2):119-124

[55] Qiu F, Lei S, Zhang L, et al. A case of nevoid basal cell carcinoma syndrome dominated by facial basal cell carcinoma. Zhong Nan Da Xue Xue Bao. Yi Xue Ban. 2022;**2022**(1672-7347):200925

[56] Glaessl A, Hohenlautner U, Landthaler M, et al. Sporadic Bazex-Dupré-Christol-like syndrome: Early onset basal cell carcinoma, hypohidrosis, hypotrichosis, and prominent milia. Dermatologic Surgery. 2000;**26**(2):152-154

[57] Atilla MK, Yllmaz Y, Bekerecioğlu M, et al. Bazex syndrome: Acrokeratosis paraneoplastica in association with simultaneous multiple genitourinary tumors. Urology. 2000;**56**(1):153

[58] Ungureanu L, Cosgarea I, Şenilă S, et al. Role of Dermoscopy in the assessment of basal cell carcinoma. Frontiers in Medicine (Lausanne). 2021;**20**(8):718855

[59] Peris K, Fargnoli MC, Garbe C, et al. European dermatology forum (EDF), the European Association of Dermato-Oncology (EADO) and the European Organization for Research and Treatment of cancer (EORTC). Diagnosis and treatment of basal cell carcinoma: European consensus-based interdisciplinary guidelines. European Journal of Cancer. 2019;**118**:10-34

[60] Zalaudek I, Moscarella E, Longo C, et al. The "signature" pattern of multiple basal cell carcinomas. Archives of Dermatology. 2012;**148**(9):1106

[61] Zhang N, Fu X, Chen X, et al. Variant subtype of xeroderma pigmentosum with multiple basal cell carcinomas diagnosed

in a Chinese woman. Photodermatology, Photoimmunology & Photomedicine. 2021;**37**(2):161-164

[62] Tiodorovic-Zivkovic D, Zalaudek I, Ferrara G, et al. Clinical and dermatoscopic findings in Bazex-Dupré-Christol and Gorlin-Goltz syndromes. Journal of the American Academy of Dermatology. 2010;**63**(4):722-724

[63] Adachi K, Yoshida Y, Noma H, et al. Characteristics of multiple basal cell carcinomas: The first study on Japanese patients. The Journal of Dermatology. 2018;**45**(10):1187-1190

[64] Savoia P, Veronese F, Camillo L, et al. Multiple basal cell carcinomas in immunocompetent patients. Cancers (Basel). 2022;**14**(13):3211

[65] Tiberio R, Valente G, Celasco M, et al. Pigmented basal cell carcinomas in Gorlin syndrome: Two cases with different dermatoscopic patterns. Clinical and Experimental Dermatology. 2011;**36**(6):617-620

[66] Niculet E, Bobeica C, Craescu M, et al. Multimodal considerations concerning basal cell carcinoma Clefting - profile of structural and aggressive traits - perspectives. Clinical, Cosmetic and Investigational Dermatology. 2022;**29**(15):2087-2095

[67] Manubens E, Barreiro A, Bennassar A, et al. Fast evaluation and monitoring of ingenol mebutate treatment of multiple basal cell carcinomas by in vivo hand-held reflectance confocal microscopy. Journal of the European Academy of Dermatology and Venereology. 2017;**31**(6):e284-e286

[68] Jerjes W, Hamdoon Z, Rashed D, et al. In vivo optical coherence tomography in assessment of suspicious facial lesions: A prospective study. Photodiagnosis and Photodynamic Therapy. 2021;**36**:102493

[69] Ho G, Schwartz RJ, Melhoranse-Gouveia B, et al. Utility of optical coherence tomography in basal cell naevus syndrome: A case report. The Australasian Journal of Dermatology. 2022;**63**(4):e331-e335

[70] Ruini C, Schuh S, Gust C, et al. Line-field optical coherence tomography: In vivo diagnosis of basal cell carcinoma subtypes compared to histopathology. Clinical and Experimental Dermatology. 2021;**46**(8):1471-1481

[71] Chuchvara N, Rao B, Liu X. Manually scanned single fiber optical coherence tomography for skin cancer characterization. Scientific Reports. 2021;**11**(1):15570

[72] Hayashi K, Okuyama R, Uhara H. Water- based correction fluid is a useful skin marker for determination of the tumor margin of basal cell carcinoma under high-frequency ultra-sound. The Journal of Dermatology. 2016;**43**(7):823-825

[73] Laverde-Saad A, Simard A, Nassim D, et al. Performance of ultrasound for identifying morphological characteristics and thickness of cutaneous basal cell carcinoma: A systematic review. Dermatology. 2022;**238**(4):692-710

[74] Khlebnikova AN, Molochkov VA, Selezneva EV, et al. Ultrasonographic features of superficial and nodular basal cell carcinoma. Medical Ultrasonography. 2018;**20**(4):475-479

[75] Aleissa S, Navarrete-Dechent C, Cordova M, et al. Presurgical evaluation of basal cell carcinoma using combined reflectance confocal microscopy-optical

coherence tomography: A prospective study. Journal of the American Academy of Dermatology. 2020;**82**(4):962-968

[76] Iftimia N, Sahu A, Cordova M, et al. The potential utility of integrated reflectance confocal microscopy-optical coherence tomography for guiding triage and therapy of basal cell carcinomas. Journal of Cancer. 2020;**11**(20):6019-6024

[77] Bilir Y, Gokce E, Ozturk B, Deresoy FA, Yuksekkaya R, Yaman E. Metastatic basal cell carcinoma accompanying gorlin syndrome. Case Reports in Oncological Medicine. 2014;**2014**:362932

[78] Saxena S, Sundaragiri KS, Bhargava A, Sankhla B. Studying the multiple faces of nevoid basal-cell carcinoma syndrome: A case series. Journal of Oral and Maxillofacial Pathology. 2020;**24**(2):315-321

[79] Berman H, Shimshak S, Reimer D, et al. Skin cancer in solid organ transplant recipients: A review for the nondermatologist. Mayo Clinic Proceedings. 2022;**97**(12):2355-2368

[80] Capasso A, Viggiano D, Lee MW, et al. Kidney transplant modifies the architecture and microenvironment of basal cell carcinomas. Kidney & Blood Pressure Research. 2020;**45**(3):368-377

[81] Madan V, Hoban P, Strange RC, Fryer AA, Lear JT. Genetics and risk factors for basal cell carcinoma. The British Journal of Dermatology. 2006;**154**(Suppl. 1):5-7

[82] Nair N, Hu Z, Du D, Gongora E. Risk prediction model for basal cell carcinoma in cardiac allograft recipients. Transplantation Proceedings. 2021;**53**(6):1981-1988

[83] Møller R, Nielsen A, Reymann F. Multiple basal cell carcinoma and internal malignant tumors. Archives of Dermatology. 1975;**111**(5):584-585

[84] Messerschmidt A, Wolter M, Ter-Nedden J, Kaufmann R, Meissner M. Multiple basal cell carcinomas arising in an epidermal nevus. Journal der Deutschen Dermatologischen Gesellschaft. 2016;**14**(11):1133-1135

[85] Kim DH, Ko HS, Jun YJ. Nonsyndromic multiple basal cell carcinomas. Archives of Craniofacial Surgery. 2017;**18**(3):191-196

[86] Zhou Q, Su W, Xu J, Lu L, Wang W. Reconstruction of multiple defects after excision of multiple basal cell carcinomas. Dermatologic Therapy. 2021;**34**(1):e14686

[87] Kim JYS, Kozlow JH, Mittal B, et al. Guidelines of care for the management of basal cell carcinoma. Journal of the American Academy of Dermatology. 2018;**78**(3):540-559

[88] Bichakjian CK, Olencki T, Aasi SZ, et al. Basal cell skin cancer, version 1.2016, NCCN clinical practice guidelines in oncology. Journal of the National Comprehensive Cancer Network. 2016;**14**(5):574-597

[89] Fournier S, Laroche A, Leblanc M, et al. Prospective clinical trial comparing curettage and cryosurgery to curettage and electrodesiccation in the management of minimally invasive basal and squamous cell carcinomas [formula: See text]. Journal of Cutaneous Medicine and Surgery. 2020;**24**(6):596-600

[90] Gross K, Kircik L, Kricorian G. 5% 5-fluorouracil cream for the treatment of small superficial basal cell carcinoma: Efficacy, tolerability, cosmetic outcome, and patient satisfaction. Dermatologic Surgery. 2007;**33**(4):433-439 discussion 440

[91] Telfer NR, Colver GB, Morton CA. Guidelines for the management of basal cell carcinoma. The British Journal of Dermatology. 2008;**159**:35-48

[92] Diluvio L, Lanna C, Lozzi F, et al. Basal cell carcinomas treated with 0.5% 5-fluorouracil and 10% salicylic acid topical solution. Dermatologic Therapy. 2019;**32**(3):e12908

[93] Naik MP, Mehta A, Abrol S, et al. Topical 5% 5-fluorouracil in the treatment of multifocal basal cell carcinoma of the face: A novel chemotherapeutic approach. Orbit-Abingdon. 2016;**35**(6):352-354

[94] Avant WH, Huff RC. Intradermal 5-fluorouracil in the treatment of basal cell carcinoma of the face. Southern Medical Journal. 1976;**69**(5):561-563

[95] Raasch B. Management of superficial basal cell carcinoma: Focus on imiquimod. Clinical, Cosmetic and Investigational Dermatology. 2009;**2**:65-75

[96] Ruiz-Villaverde R, Sánchez-Cano D, Burkhardt-Pérez P. Superficial basal cell carcinoma treated with imiquimod 5% topical cream for a 4-week period: A case series. Journal of the European Academy of Dermatology and Venereology. 2009;**23**(7):828-831

[97] Marks R, Gebauer K, Shumack S, et al. Imiquimod 5% cream in the treatment of superficial basal cell carcinoma: Results of a multicenter 6-week dose-response trial. Journal of the American Academy of Dermatology. 2001;**44**(5):807-813

[98] Jansen MHE, Mosterd K, Arits AHMM, et al. Five-year results of a randomized controlled trial comparing effectiveness of photodynamic therapy, topical imiquimod, and topical 5-fluorouracil in patients with superficial basal cell carcinoma. The Journal of Investigative Dermatology. 2017;**138**(3):527-533

[99] Micali G, Lacarrubba F, Nasca MR, et al. The use of imiquimod 5% cream for the treatment of basal cell carcinoma as observed in Gorlin's syndrome. Clinical and Experimental Dermatology. 2003;**28**(Suppl. 1):19-23

[100] Drehs MM, Cook-Bolden F, Tanzi EL, et al. Successful treatment of multiple superficial basal cell carcinomas with topical imiquimod: Case report and review of the literature. Dermatologic Surgery. 2002;**28**(5):427-429

[101] Marks R, Owens M, Walters SA. Efficacy and safety of 5% imiquimod cream in treating patients with multiple superficial basal cell carcinomas. Archives of Dermatology. 2004;**140**(10):1284-1285

[102] Yu Y, Zhang G, Fu S. Comprehensive treatment of basal cell carcinoma in nevoid basal cell carcinoma syndrome with 5-fluorouracil and salicylic acid. Dermatologic Therapy. 2022;**35**(12):e15972

[103] Glass LF, Jaroszeski M, Gilbert R, et al. Intralesional bleomycin-mediated electrochemotherapy in 20 patients with basal cell carcinoma. Journal of the American Academy of Dermatology. 1997;**37**(4):596-599

[104] Gyurova MS, Stancheva MZ, Arnaudova MN, Yankova RK. Intralesional bleomycin as alternative therapy in the treatment of multiple basal cell carcinomas. Dermatology Online Journal. 2006;**12**(3):25

[105] Cooper SM, Dawber RP. The history of cryosurgery. Journal of the Royal Society of Medicine. 2001;**94**(4):196-201

[106] Tsuji T, Otake N, Nishimura M. Cryosurgery and topical fluorouracil: A treatment method for widespread basal cell epithelioma in basal cell nevus syndrome. The Journal of Dermatology. 1993;**20**(8):507-513

[107] Lindgren G, Larkö O. Cryosurgery of eyelid basal cell carcinomas including 781 cases treated over 30 years. Acta Ophthalmologica. 2014;**92**:787-792

[108] Lindemalm-Lundstam B, Dalenbäck J. Prospective follow-up after curettage-cryosurgery for scalp and face skin cancers. The British Journal of Dermatology. 2009;**161**:568-576

[109] Nordin P, Larko O, Stenquist B. Five-year results of curettage-cryosurgery of selected large primary basal cell carcinomas on the nose: An alternative treatment in a geographical area underserved by Mohs' surgery. The British Journal of Dermatology. 1997;**136**(2):180-183

[110] Nordin P, Stenquist B. Five-year results of curettage-cryosurgery for 100 consecutive auricular non-melanoma skin cancers. The Journal of Laryngology and Otology. 2002;**116**(11):893-898

[111] Backman EJ, Polesie S, Berglund S, et al. Curettage vs. cryosurgery for superficial basal cell carcinoma: A prospective, randomised and controlled trial. Journal of the European Academy of Dermatology and Venereology. 2022;**36**(10):1758-1765

[112] Tchanque-Fossuo CN, Eisen DB. A systematic review on the use of cryotherapy versus other treatments for basal cell carcinoma. Dermatology Online Journal. 2018;**24**(11):13030/qt49k1c38t

[113] Rizzo JM, Segal RJ, Zeitouni NC. Combination vismodegib and photodynamic therapy for multiple basal cell carcinomas. Photodiagnosis and Photodynamic Therapy. 2018;**21**:58-62

[114] Li C, Chen P, Li Z, et al. 5-aminolevulinic acid photodynamic therapy and excision surgery for nevoid basal cell carcinoma syndrome with multiple basal cell carcinomas and PTCH1 mutation. Photodiagnosis and Photodynamic Therapy. 2020;**32**:101968

[115] Liao C, Zhang G, Wang P, Sun X, Wang X. Combination curettage and modified ALA-PDT for multiple basal cell carcinomas of the face and head. Photodiagnosis and Photodynamic Therapy. 2021;**35**:102393

[116] Cao D, Zhu W, Kuang Y, Zhao S. A safe and effective treatment: Surgery combined with photodynamic therapy for multiple basal cell carcinomas. Photodiagnosis and Photodynamic Therapy. 2019;**28**:133-135

[117] Sorensen A, Wolter S, Patel N, et al. Dermoscopy for identification of basal cell carcinomas in basal cell nevus syndrome during carbon dioxide laser surgery. Pediatric Dermatology. 2016;**33**(1):109-111

[118] Chen GS, Yu HS, Lan CC, et al. CXC chemokine receptor CXCR4 expression enhances tumorigenesis and angiogenesis of basal cell carcinoma. The British Journal of Dermatology. 2006;**154**(5):910-918

[119] Anderson RR, Parrish JA. Selective photothermolysis: Precise microsurgery by selective absorption of pulsed radiation. Science. 1983;**220**(4596):524-527

[120] Campolmi P, Troiano M, Bonan P, Cannarozzo G, Lotti T. Vascular based non conventional dye laser treatment for basal cell carcinoma. Dermatologic Therapy. 2008;**21**(5):402-405

[121] Shah SM, Konnikov N, Duncan LM, et al. The effect of 595nm pulsed dye laser on superficial and nodular basal cell carcinomas. Lasers in Surgery and Medicine. 2009;**41**(6):417-422

[122] Marous M, Mueller K, Tausk F. Multiple basal cell carcinomas in Gorlin syndrome treated with pulsed dye laser. Journal of Cosmetic and Laser Therapy. 2020;**22**(6-8):230-231

[123] Aszterbaum M, Epstein J, Oro A, et al. Ultraviolet and ionizing radiation enhance the growth of BCCs and trichoblastomas in patched heterozygous knockout mice. Nature Medicine. 1999;**5**(11):1285-1291

[124] Frentz G, Munch-Petersen B, Wulf HC, et al. The nevoid basal cell carcinoma syndrome: Sensitivity to ultraviolet and x-ray irradiation. Journal of the American Academy of Dermatology. 1987;**17**(4):637-643

[125] Strong LC. Genetic and environmental interactions. Cancer. 1977;**40**(4 Suppl):1861-1866

[126] Baker S, Joseph K, Tai P. Radiotherapy in Gorlin syndrome: Can it be safe and effective in adult patients? Journal of Cutaneous Medicine and Surgery. 2016;**20**(2):159-162

[127] Caccialanza M, Percivalle S, Piccinno R. Possibility of treating basal cell carcinomas of nevoid basal cell carcinoma syndrome with superficial x-ray therapy. Dermatology. 2004;**208**(1):60-63

[128] Ron E, Preston DL, Kishikawa M, et al. Skin tumor risk among atomic-bomb survivors in Japan. Cancer Causes & Control. 1998;**9**:393-401

[129] Karagas MR, McDonald J, Greenberg E, et al. Risk of basal cell and squamous cell skin cancers after ionizing radiation therapy. Journal of the National Cancer Institute. 1996;**88**:1848-1853

[130] Ciążyńska M, Narbutt J, Skibińska M, et al. Itraconazole-a new player in the therapy of advanced basal cell carcinoma: A case report. JCO Oncology Practice. 2020;**16**(12):837-838

[131] Cosio T, Di Prete M, Campione E. Arsenic trioxide, Itraconazole, all-trans retinoic acid and nicotinamide: A proof of concept for combined treatments with hedgehog inhibitors in advanced basal cell carcinoma. Biomedicine. 2020;**8**(6):156

[132] Kim DJ, Kim J, Spaunhurst K, et al. Open-label, exploratory phase II trial of oral itraconazole for the treatment of basal cell carcinoma. Journal of Clinical Oncology. 2014;**32**(8):745-751

[133] Kim J, Aftab BT, Tang JY, et al. Itraconazole and arsenic trioxide inhibit hedgehog pathway activation and tumor growth associated with acquired resistance to smoothened antagonists. Cancer Cell. 2013;**23**(1):23-34

[134] Ogden SK, Ascano M Jr, Stegman MA, et al. Regulation of hedgehog signaling: A complex story. Biochemical Pharmacology. 2004;**67**(5):805-814

[135] Eibenschutz L, Caputo S, Camera E, et al. Evaluation of hedgehog pathway inhibition on nevoid basal cell carcinoma syndrome fibroblasts and basal cell carcinoma-associated fibroblasts: Are Vismodegib and Sonidegib useful to target cancer-prone fibroblasts? Cancers (Basel). 2021;**13**(22):5858

[136] Gambini D, Passoni E, Nazzaro G, et al. Basal cell carcinoma and hedgehog pathway inhibitors: Focus on immune response. Frontiers in Medicine (Lausanne). 2022;**9**:893063

[137] Zargari O, Azimi SZ, Geranmayeh S. Inoperable infiltrative basal cell carcinoma successfully treated with vismodegib. Dermatologic Therapy. 2017;**30**(4):10.1111/dth.12509

[138] Migden M, Farberg AS, Dummer R, et al. A review of hedgehog inhibitors Sonidegib and Vismodegib for treatment of advanced basal cell carcinoma. Journal of Drugs in Dermatology. 2021;**20**(2):156-165

[139] Niebel D, Sirokay J, Hoffmann F, et al. Clinical management of locally advanced basal-cell carcinomas and future therapeutic directions. Dermatology and Therapy. 2020;**10**(4):835-846

Section 3

# Alternative Therapy for BCC

Chapter 5

# Radiation Therapy for Basal Cell Skin Cancer

*Eter Natelauri and Anna Jghamadze*


## Abstract

Radiation therapy significantly treats basal cell carcinoma (BCC), offering effective tumor control and favorable cosmetic outcomes. Basal cell carcinoma is the most common form of skin cancer, and radiation therapy is indicated in cases where surgery is not feasible or for high-risk features. External beam radiation therapy, brachytherapy, proton therapy, and electronic brachytherapy are the treatment modalities employed in BCC management. Tumor control rates with radiation therapy for BCC are generally high, with excellent local control achieved. Toxicities associated with radiation therapy for BCC include acute effects on the skin and adjacent structures, such as radiation dermatitis and hair loss. Minimizing toxicities and optimizing patient comfort involve advanced treatment planning techniques, appropriate skin care, and supportive care measures. Ongoing clinical trials and future perspectives in radiation therapy for BCC focus on targeted therapies, immunotherapies, hypofractionation, and advanced radiation techniques. These research efforts aim to improve treatment outcomes, personalize therapy, and enhance patient satisfaction. This chapter provides a concise overview of radiation therapy for BCC, highlighting its indications, techniques, outcomes, toxicities, and future perspectives.


**Keywords:** radiation therapy, basal cell skin cancer, tumor control, cosmetic outcomes, indications, techniques, outcomes, toxicities, future perspectives, clinical trials, targeted therapies, immunotherapies, hypofractionation, advanced radiation techniques

## 1. Introduction

Skin cancer is one of the most prevalent forms worldwide, with its incidence steadily increasing over the years [1]. Basal cell carcinoma (BCC) is the most commonly diagnosed among the various types of skin cancer, accounting for approximately 80% of all cases [2]. While BCC is generally characterized by slow growth and low metastatic potential, it can lead to a significant local invasion, causing substantial morbidity and cosmetic concerns for affected individuals. Therefore, effective treatment modalities are crucial to achieving optimal outcomes in patients with BCC.

Radiation therapy (RT) has emerged as a valuable and versatile treatment option for managing BCC, particularly when surgical intervention may be challenging or undesirable. Radiation therapy utilizes high-energy ionizing radiation to target and destroy cancer cells while minimizing damage to surrounding healthy tissues. In the early 1900s, radiation was first used to treat a patient suffering from skin cancer. As advances were made in dermatology and surgical procedures, the importance of radiation therapy in treating skin cancer decreased significantly over time [3]. However, there are still some circumstances in which radiation therapy has advantages over alternative treatment techniques that are now available. Over the years, radiation therapy techniques and protocols for BCC have also evolved, allowing for more precise and effective treatment delivery [4].

To establish a foundation for understanding radiation therapy for BCC, it is essential to delve into the pathogenesis and clinical characteristics of basal cell carcinoma. BCC arises from the abnormal growth of basal cells located in the epidermis's lower layer. Various subtypes of BCC, such as nodular, infiltrative, and morpheaform variants, present distinct clinical features and implications for treatment selection. Understanding these subtypes is critical for tailoring radiation therapy approaches to individual patients. The decision to employ radiation therapy for BCC is often driven by specific clinical scenarios where radiation therapy may be preferred over surgical excision. These scenarios include primary BCCs located in anatomically challenging areas, cases of recurrent BCC, large or high-risk BCCs, and situations where patients have contraindications to surgery. By exploring these indications, healthcare professionals can understand when radiation therapy may offer optimal results and improved patient outcomes. Clinical outcomes play a significant role in evaluating the efficacy of radiation therapy for BCC. Healthcare professionals can refine treatment strategies and optimize patient care by identifying factors influencing treatment outcomes. The use of adjuvant radiation therapy following surgical excision or in combination with other treatment modalities, such as topical therapies or immunomodulatory agents, will also be explored. By understanding the acute and late effects on the skin, adjacent structures, and surrounding tissues, healthcare professionals can implement strategies to minimize these toxicities and enhance patient comfort during and after treatment.

## 2. Basal cell carcinoma: pathogenesis and clinical characteristics

Basal cell carcinoma (BCC) is the most common type of skin cancer, originating from the basal cells that line the deepest layer of the epidermis. It predominantly affects body areas exposed to ultraviolet (UV) radiation, such as the face, neck, and arms. BCC typically grows slowly and rarely spreads to other body parts, making it highly curable if detected and treated early. There are several subtypes of Basal Cell Carcinoma [5]:

- The superficial subtype of basal cell carcinoma (BCC) is characterized by multiple tiny buds of basaloid cells extending from the epidermis without invading the dermis.

- The nodular variant is the most common type of BCC. It consists of cell clusters arranged in islands with peripheral palisading, while the central cells show a haphazard arrangement. Larger nodular BCCs may exhibit ulceration.

- The micronodular subtype shares histologic similarities with the nodular subtype but comprises multiple small nodules. The micronodular type has a higher risk of local recurrence than other subtypes.

- The sclerosing (morphea-like) subtype is characterized by spiky, basaloid strands of cells invading the dermis, surrounded by dense fibrous tissue. The differential diagnosis may consider microcystic adnexal carcinoma, desmoplastic trichoepithelioma, or metastatic cancer due to similar histologic features. In cases where the tumor nests exhibit spiky projections and invade deeply, it is called an infiltrative BCC.

- Pigmented BCC occurs when melanocytes and melanin are present alongside the tumor cells. This subtype is more frequently observed in the superficial, micronodular, or follicular variants.

- The infundibulocystic variant is a rare subtype often found on the face. It manifests as a well-defined tumor composed of cell nests arranged in an anastomosing manner with minimal stromal involvement. Numerous small infundibular cyst-like structures containing keratinous material and occasionally melanin can be observed.

- Basosquamous or metatypical BCC exhibits BCC and squamous cell carcinoma (SCC) features. The exact nature of this lesion is debated, but it typically refers to a rare form of BCC characterized by nests and strands of cells that mature into more extensive and paler cells without peripheral palisading.

- Fibroepithelioma of Pinkus appears as a soft nodular lesion resembling a fibroma or papilloma commonly found on the lower back. It consists of interconnected strands and aggregates of basaloid cells surrounded by fibrous stroma.

The clinical presentation of BCC can vary depending on the subtype. Common signs include pearly or translucent appearance; raised, firm, or shiny nodules; ulceration, crusting, or bleeding; slow growth and lack of pain or itchiness; telangiectasia (visible blood vessels); and distorted or rolled borders.

Diagnostic approaches for basal cell skin cancer (BCC) typically involve a combination of clinical examination, dermatoscopic evaluation, and biopsy procedures. These approaches aim to identify and characterize the BCC lesion accurately, guiding appropriate treatment decisions. Here are the critical diagnostic approaches:

- Clinical Examination: A dermatologist conducts a thorough visual examination of the skin, looking for characteristic signs of BCC. These signs may include a raised, pearly bump with a rolled border, small blood vessels on the surface (telangiectasia), central ulceration or crusting, and slow growth over time. The examination may involve assessing the lesion's size, shape, color, and associated symptoms.

- Dermatoscopy: Dermatoscopy, also known as dermoscopy or epiluminescence microscopy, is a noninvasive technique that uses a dermatoscope—a handheld magnifying device with a light source—to examine the skin lesion in detail [6]. Dermatoscopy allows the dermatologist to visualize specific patterns and structures within the lesion, helping to differentiate BCC from other skin conditions.

- Biopsy: Biopsy is the gold standard diagnostic procedure for BCC. It involves the removal of a small sample of tissue from the suspicious lesion for microscopic examination by a pathologist. Different biopsy techniques can be used depending on the size, location, and clinical features of the lesion:

- Shave Biopsy: A superficial lesion sample is shaved off using a scalpel or a razor blade.
- Punch Biopsy: A circular tool removes a small, full-thickness sample of the lesion, including the epidermis and part of the dermis.
- Excisional Biopsy: The entire lesion and a margin of surrounding healthy tissue are surgically excised and sent for examination.
- Incisional Biopsy: Only a representative portion of the lesion is surgically excised and examined.

The biopsy sample is sent to a pathology laboratory, where it is processed, stained, and examined under a microscope by a pathologist. The microscopic analysis helps confirm BCC's presence, determine the subtype (e.g., nodular, superficial, or infiltrative), and assess essential features such as depth of invasion and aggressive characteristics.

In some cases, additional diagnostic techniques may be used for specific scenarios:

- Imaging Techniques: In rare cases where the BCC may have invaded deeper structures, imaging techniques such as ultrasound, computed tomography (CT), or magnetic resonance imaging (MRI) can provide valuable information about tumor depth and involvement of underlying structures and aid in treatment planning.
- Molecular Testing: Molecular testing, such as genetic analysis or immunohistochemistry, may be employed when the diagnosis is challenging or when determining treatment options, particularly for rare or aggressive subtypes of BCC.

It is important to note that diagnosis and treatment decisions are best made by a qualified healthcare professional, such as a dermatologist, based on clinical evaluation, dermatoscopy, biopsy results, and individual patient factors [7].

The clinical characteristics and subtypes of BCC have implications for treatment selection. Factors such as tumor size, location, depth of invasion, and histological subtype influence the choice of treatment modality. While surgical excision is the standard approach for most BCCs, radiation therapy is crucial in cases where surgery may be challenging or associated with significant morbidity. Understanding the specific characteristics of BCC subtypes aids in tailoring treatment plans and achieving optimal patient outcomes.

By comprehending BCC's pathogenesis and clinical characteristics, healthcare professionals can accurately recognize and diagnose the disease. This knowledge is the foundation for selecting appropriate treatment strategies, including radiation therapy, that effectively address basal cell carcinoma's unique features and challenges.

## 3. Indications for radiation therapy in basal cell skin cancer

Radiation therapy (RT) is a valuable treatment modality for basal cell carcinoma (BCC), offering an effective alternative or complementary approach to surgical excision. While surgery remains the primary treatment for most BCC cases, there are specific clinical scenarios where radiation therapy becomes a preferred or necessary option [8]. Understanding these indications is crucial for healthcare professionals in determining the optimal treatment approach for patients with BCC.

A. Primary BCCs in Challenging Anatomical Areas

- Periocular and Periorbital BCCs: BCCs located near the eyes or in delicate anatomical regions pose challenges for surgical excision due to the potential for functional and cosmetic complications. Radiation therapy can be an effective treatment option for preserving visual function and achieving satisfactory cosmetic outcomes.

- Nasal and Facial BCCs: BCCs involving the nose and other facial regions often require complex reconstruction after surgical removal, which can be technically demanding. Radiation therapy can be considered an alternative or adjunctive treatment, particularly in cases where surgical excision compromises the functional and esthetic integrity of the nose or surrounding structures.

- Ear BCCs: The ears are susceptible to BCC development, and surgical excision in this area can lead to deformities and functional impairment. Radiation therapy can be employed as a primary treatment or as an adjuvant therapy to surgical excision to preserve the structural and functional integrity of the ears.

B. Recurrent BCCs

- BCC's recurrence after initial treatment can present challenges in managing the disease effectively. Radiation therapy offers a valuable option for recurrent BCCs, especially if previous surgical excisions have been unsuccessful or if the tumor recurs in anatomically challenging areas where further surgeries may not be feasible or desirable.

C. Large or High-Risk BCCs

- Large BCCs: Large BCCs, typically those exceeding 2 cm in diameter, present challenges in complete surgical removal while preserving optimal cosmetic outcomes. Radiation therapy can be employed as the primary treatment or in combination with surgical excision to achieve tumor control and maintain cosmesis.

- High-Risk BCCs: Certain BCCs have a higher risk of recurrences or aggressive behavior, such as infiltrative or morpheaform subtypes, tumors with aggressive histological features, or those located in functionally or cosmetically critical areas. Radiation therapy may be utilized as a definitive or adjuvant therapy to reduce the risk of recurrence and improve local control in high-risk BCCs.

- Contraindications to Surgery: In some cases, patients may have contraindications to surgical excisions, such as underlying medical conditions or anatomical factors that make surgery risky or impractical. Radiation therapy can be an effective alternative, providing a noninvasive treatment option for BCCs while minimizing surgical risks and complications.

By understanding the indications for radiation therapy in BCC, healthcare professionals can make informed treatment decisions based on individual patient factors, tumor characteristics, and radiation therapy's potential benefits and limitations. Collaborative decision-making between healthcare providers and patients is essential to determine the most suitable treatment approach that maximizes outcomes while considering patient preferences and overall health.

## 4. Technical aspects of radiation therapy for basal cell skin cancer

Effective treatment planning is crucial for achieving optimal outcomes in radiation therapy (RT) for basal cell carcinoma (BCC). Careful consideration of various factors helps develop individualized treatment plans targeting the tumor while minimizing radiation exposure to surrounding healthy tissues [9]. The following treatment planning considerations are essential in the context of RT for BCC:

Pretreatment Evaluation:

- Clinical Assessment: A thorough clinical evaluation is essential to determine the tumor size, location, and characteristics accurately. Precise tumor delineation is critical for treatment planning.

- Imaging Studies: Imaging modalities such as computed tomography (CT) or magnetic resonance imaging (MRI) may be employed to assess tumor depth and the invasion of adjacent structures and identify potential lymph node involvement.

Radiation Technique Selection:

- External Beam Radiation Therapy (EBRT): EBRT involves delivering radiation from a machine outside the body, focusing radiation beams to the tumor site. Techniques such as 3D conformal radiation therapy (3D-CRT), intensity-modulated radiation therapy (IMRT), or volumetric modulated arc therapy (VMAT) may be used to optimize dose distribution and spare healthy tissues.

- Brachytherapy: Brachytherapy involves the placement of radioactive sources directly into or near the tumor site. This technique can be utilized in cases where the tumor is superficial or in difficult-to-treat areas, allowing for a highly targeted and localized radiation dose.

- Proton Therapy: Proton therapy utilizes protons instead of conventional X-ray photons, providing superior dose conformity and sparing surrounding healthy tissues. It may be considered for some instances of BCC, particularly in pediatric patients or those with complex tumor geometries.

- Electronic Brachytherapy: Electronic brachytherapy employs low-energy X-rays from a portable device, allowing for targeted treatment of superficial BCCs. It offers a noninvasive and convenient option for patients, especially in cases where traditional brachytherapy is not feasible.

Treatment Field Design:

- Tumor Volume Definition: Precise delineation of the target volume is crucial to ensure accurate radiation delivery. The gross tumor volume (GTV), clinical target volume (CTV), and planning target volume (PTV) should be carefully defined based on clinical assessment and imaging studies.

- Margin Considerations: Adequate margins are added around the GTV to account for treatment delivery, patient setup, and organ motion uncertainties. Advanced imaging techniques, such as 4D CT, can aid in accounting for respiratory motion and further refining the treatment margins.

- Organ-at-Risk (OAR) Constraints: Critical structures near the tumor, such as the eyes, optic nerves, lens, brainstem, spinal cord, and skin, must be carefully considered to minimize radiation-related toxicity. Dose constraints and dose-volume histogram (DVH) analysis helps ensure that the dose limits to OARs are not exceeded.

Dose Fractionation:

- Standard Fractionation: The most commonly used dose fractionation schedule for BCC is delivering a total dose of 60–70 Gray (Gy) in daily fractions of 2 Gy over several weeks (e.g., 6–7 weeks) [8].

- Hypofractionation: Hypofractionated schedules may be considered in exceptional cases, delivering higher doses per fraction with fewer treatment sessions. These schedules can be completed in a shorter overall treatment time, enhancing patient convenience.

## 5. External beam radiation therapy

External beam radiation therapy (EBRT) is widely used in treating basal cell carcinoma (BCC). It involves delivering radiation to the tumor site using a machine outside the body. EBRT offers precise and targeted radiation delivery, allowing for effective tumor control while minimizing radiation exposure to surrounding healthy tissues.

Prior to treatment, a simulation session is conducted to obtain images of the patient's treatment area. Imaging modalities such as CT or MRI scans provide detailed information about the tumor and surrounding structures, aiding in treatment planning. Appropriate immobilization devices, such as thermoplastic masks or body molds, ensure consistent positioning during treatment sessions. Immobilization devices help minimize patient movement, allowing for accurate radiation delivery.

Target Volume Delineation: The gross tumor volume (GTV) and clinical target volume (CTV) are defined based on clinical assessment, imaging data, and surgical scars if present. The planning target volume (PTV) is then generated by adding appropriate margins around the CTV to account for treatment setup and patient motion uncertainties. The radiation therapy (RT) target volume or field is determined by factors such as lesion size, location, and growth type. Infiltrative lesions, which require more extensive coverage, have larger field margins. Typically, the treatment field encompasses the visible or palpable tumor and approximately 1 cm to 2 cm of surrounding normal-appearing skin [8]. In cases where the lesion is well-demarcated and measures 1 cm or smaller, tighter margins of 1 cm may be used, especially when treating areas near the eye. However, lesions with ill-defined borders necessitate more generous margins to include subclinical microscopic extensions adequately.

In patients receiving postoperative RT for lymph node metastasis or perineural invasion (PNI), the initial portal may need to include the primary tumor bed if technically feasible. However, this inclusion may be omitted if more than 12 months have passed since treatment at the primary site, with no evidence of local recurrence. Some clinicians may extend this period, such as waiting for 24 months, before omitting treatment at the primary site.

Determining the clinical target volume in PNI depends on the specific primary site and the cranial nerves involved. In many cases, this includes areas such as the skull base, cavernous sinus, and intracranial routes back to the brainstem. Advanced techniques such as highly conformal intensity-modulated radiation therapy (IMRT) or intensity-modulated proton therapy (IMPT) enable precise treatment of neural pathways while minimizing radiation exposure to critical structures. Therefore, clinicians must possess sufficient knowledge and expertise when delineating the relevant structures. This ensures the accurate delivery of radiation therapy while preserving normal tissue function [10]. Elective treatment of regional lymph nodes in patients with PNI is an option, but its benefit has yet to be established or proven. The decision to include regional lymph nodes in the treatment plan should be carefully evaluated and individualized based on the specific clinical scenario and available evidence.

Advanced treatment planning systems are utilized to optimize dose distribution and ensure adequate coverage of the target while sparing nearby critical structures. Techniques such as 3D conformal radiation therapy (3D-CRT), intensity-modulated radiation therapy (IMRT), or volumetric modulated arc therapy (VMAT) may be employed to achieve desired dose distributions. For treatment with X-rays, the dose is specified at Dmax (maximum dose). In contrast, when irradiating with electrons, the dose is typically prescribed at 90% of the specified dose. This distinction accounts for the differences in the relative biologic effectiveness between these two types of radiation beams. Structures, including the eyes, optic nerves, lens, brainstem, spinal cord, and skin, are carefully delineated and considered during treatment planning. Dose constraints are established to minimize radiation-related toxicity to these structures.

The total prescribed dose for BCC is typically delivered in daily fractions over several weeks. The standard fractionation scheme is 2 Gy per fraction, delivered 5 days per week, resulting in a total 60–70 Gy dose. In exceptional cases, hypofractionated schedules may be considered, delivering higher doses per fraction with fewer treatment sessions. The recommended radiation regimen for individual patients depends on several factors, including patient age, performance status, lesion size, and site. For older patients aged 60 to 80 years, a dose of 40 Gy in 10 fractions, 45 Gy in 15 fractions, or 50–55 Gy in 20–25 fractions is considered appropriate and effective.

In cases where patients are elderly (over 80 years of age) and/or in poor general condition, hypofractionation may be utilized. Hypofractionation involves delivering a lower total dose of radiation in more significant fractions, such as 32 Gy in 4 fractions, 21 Gy in 3 fractions, 35 Gy in 5 fractions, or a single dose of 15 to 20 Gy. Despite the use of hypofractionation, excellent control rates are still expected. However, it should be noted that delivering more significant fractions using superficial energy photons or orthovoltage energy photons may take longer (20 to 30 minutes), and uncooperative patients may require light sedation. Numerous studies have shown that hypofractionated radiation therapy achieves over 90% local control rates with limited side effects [11].

In cases where a nodal basin (such as the parotid or neck) has been surgically resected and multiple positive nodes or a single node with extranodal spread are present, patients usually receive radiation in 2 Gy fractions to a total dose of 60 Gy due to the more extensive treatment volume involved. Similarly, for patients with inoperable nodal disease who are treated with radiation therapy alone, fractions of 2 to 2.5 Gy are administered, with a total dose ranging from 60 to 70 Gy, unless the intent of treatment is solely palliative.

Before each treatment session, patient positioning is verified using image guidance techniques, such as cone-beam CT or portal imaging. This ensures accurate alignment with the planned treatment position, minimizing setup errors. High-energy X-ray beams generated by linear accelerators (linacs) are commonly used in EBRT for BCC. The choice of beam energy and beam angles depends on the tumor location, depth, and nearby critical structures. Beam modulation techniques, such as dynamic multileaf collimation in IMRT or VMAT, allow for precise shaping of the radiation dose to conform to the tumor shape while sparing healthy tissues.

Regular treatment reviews and quality assurance procedures are performed throughout the course to ensure accurate and consistent radiation delivery. Patients undergoing EBRT for BCC require regular follow-up visits to monitor treatment response, assess acute side effects, and manage potential late effects. Collaboration between radiation oncologists, dermatologists, and other healthcare professionals is essential in providing comprehensive patient care.

External beam radiation therapy plays a significant role in treating BCC, especially in cases where surgical excision may be challenging or associated with significant morbidity. By carefully considering treatment simulation, planning, delivery techniques, and monitoring treatment, healthcare professionals can effectively utilize EBRT to achieve optimal tumor control while minimizing radiation-related toxicity for patients with BCC.

## 6. Brachytherapy techniques

Brachytherapy is a radiation therapy technique that involves the placement of radioactive sources directly into or near the tumor site. It provides a highly targeted and localized radiation dose, making it an effective treatment option for basal cell carcinoma (BCC), particularly in cases where the tumor is superficial or in difficult-to-treat areas. Brachytherapy offers several advantages, including precise dose delivery, reduced treatment duration, and sparing of surrounding healthy tissues. Various brachytherapy techniques can be employed for the treatment of BCC:

- Surface Brachytherapy/Electronic Brachytherapy: Electronic brachytherapy, also known as low-energy or superficial brachytherapy, utilizes low-energy X-rays emitted from a portable device. It is commonly used for superficial BCCs, delivering radiation directly to the skin surface. This technique offers a noninvasive and convenient option for patients, especially in cases where traditional brachytherapy is not feasible. Applicators specifically designed for flat surfaces eliminate the need for anesthesia during application. These applicators, including French pulmonary applicators, can treat skin surface lesions. Once the applicator is prepared, markers are inserted into the catheters to simulate the presence of the radioactive source. X-rays (front-rear and lateral) or computed tomography (CT) scans are performed to gather imaging data, which are then transferred to the planning system. During the planning stage, the area to be irradiated, known as the planning target volume (PTV), consists of the tumor along with a margin of either 0.5 or 1 cm (known as the gross tumor volume - GTV), depending on the diameter of the lesion [12, 13]. As per the recommendations of the American Brachytherapy Society, tumors with an infiltration depth of less than 0.5 cm can be treated solely with superficial brachytherapy (BT). The suggested dose for this approach is 48–51 Gy delivered in 16–17 fractions, with the treatment extending 0.5 cm from the surface of the applicator. This treatment is administered once daily [14].

- Contact Brachytherapy: Contact brachytherapy involves placing a radioactive source, such as a surface mold or applicator, directly on the skin surface. The source remains in contact with the tumor site for a specified duration, delivering radiation to the target area while minimizing exposure to surrounding healthy tissues.

- Interstitial Brachytherapy/Needle- or Catheter-Based Brachytherapy: Interstitial brachytherapy involves the insertion of radioactive sources directly into the tumor or surrounding tissues using needles or catheters. This technique allows for the precise placement of radiation sources at specific depths and positions within the tumor, tailoring the dose distribution to the tumor volume. Tumors situated on curved surfaces such as naso-buccal folds, fingers, and ear pinna, with a diameter ranging from 5 to 6 cm and a thickness of 0.5 to 2.0 cm, are best treated using interstitial brachytherapy (BT). Cases involving coexisting fistula, nodal metastasis, and bone infiltration are not considered in this context. Typically, 1 to 3 plastic applicators are implanted into the tumor, and a prescribed dose of 65 Gy (ranging from 45 to 70 Gy) is calculated for the reference isodoses of 85% according to the Paris system. These procedures have shown significant benefits in achieving local control rates ranging from 95–98% while preserving excellent cosmetic and functional outcomes [15]. In the interstitial method, some centers still employ hypodermic needles with bevels of 2 to 10 cm in length, along with silk and nylon wire tubes adapted for afterloading applications. Local or general anesthesia is administered as needed during these procedures.

- Similarly, metal applicators are used for the interstitial implantation of radioactive iridium wires with a thickness of 0.5 cm. The number of applicators or needles required depends on the diameter of the tumor; for most skin cancers infiltrating healthy tissues by less than 1 cm, single-plane high-dose-rate (HDR) applications are performed. Standard dose regimens for T1–2 tumors typically involve 48 Gy delivered in 16 fractions administered twice daily. For T3–4 tumors, the standard dose is 51 Gy, delivered in 17 fractions, also given twice daily [16].

- High-Dose Rate (HDR) Brachytherapy: HDR brachytherapy delivers a high dose of radiation over a short period, typically in fractions delivered a few times a day. It involves temporarily placing radioactive sources in the tumor site using afterloading techniques. The sources are remotely controlled, allowing for precise dose delivery and flexibility in treatment planning.

- Seed Implantation/Permanent Seed Implantation: Permanent seed implantation involves the placement of tiny, radioactive seeds directly into the tumor. These seeds emit radiation over an extended period, gradually delivering the prescribed dose. This technique is typically used for low-risk or small BCCs and allows continuous dose delivery while minimizing treatment sessions.

Multimodal Approaches:

Brachytherapy with EBRT: Brachytherapy can be combined with EBRT to achieve optimal treatment outcomes. EBRT delivers radiation to the tumor site from outside the body, while brachytherapy provides a boost dose to the tumor area [17]. This combination approach allows for better coverage of the target volume while sparing surrounding healthy tissues.

During brachytherapy treatment planning for BCC, imaging studies, such as CT or MRI scans, precisely delineate the tumor volume and surrounding structures. Treatment optimization is performed to ensure adequate target dose coverage while minimizing radiation exposure to critical structures. Close collaboration between radiation oncologists, medical physicists, and dosimetrists is essential in determining each patient's optimal brachytherapy technique and dose distribution [18].

Brachytherapy techniques provide an effective and localized treatment option for BCC, particularly in cases where surgical excision may be challenging or result in functional or cosmetic complications. The selection of the appropriate brachytherapy technique depends on factors such as tumor characteristics, size, location, and patient-specific considerations. By employing these techniques, healthcare professionals can achieve precise tumor control while preserving the quality of life for patients with BCC.

## 7. Proton therapy

PT is a specialized form of EBRT that utilizes protons, rather than conventional X-ray photons, to deliver radiation to the tumor site [19]. Protons have unique physical properties that allow for precise dose deposition, resulting in superior dose conformity and sparing of healthy tissues compared to photon-based treatments. PT offers the advantage of utilizing the finite range of protons, which allows for the sparing of healthy tissue from receiving beam exit doses that would otherwise be exposed in photon-based treatments. However, the current evidence on PT for skin cancer is limited to comparative dosimetric analyses and retrospective single-institution series. However, proton therapy may be considered for some basal cell carcinoma (BCC) instances, particularly in pediatric patients or those with complex tumor geometries.

Advantages of Proton Therapy for BCC:

- Superior Dose Conformity: Proton beams have a characteristic Bragg peak, where the most radiation dose is deposited at a specific depth within the tumor. This allows for highly conformal dose distributions, minimizing radiation exposure to surrounding healthy tissues.

- Reduced Radiation to Critical Structures: Proton therapy can spare critical structures near the tumor, such as the eyes, optic nerves, and brainstem. This is particularly advantageous in BCC cases where the tumor is in close proximity to these critical structures.

- Reduced Risk of Late Effects: The precise dose deposition of proton therapy can reduce the risk of long-term radiation-related side effects, enhancing the quality of life for BCC patients after treatment.

Considerations for Proton Therapy in BCC:

- Tumor Characteristics: Proton therapy may be considered for BCC cases with challenging tumor locations, complex geometries, or tumors in close proximity to critical structures where conventional radiation techniques may pose a higher risk of complications.

- Availability and Access: Proton therapy facilities are currently limited in number and may not be readily accessible to all patients. Referral to specialized centers and multidisciplinary collaboration is essential in determining the suitability of proton therapy for individual cases.

Proton therapy offers unique advantages in treating BCC, providing tailored radiation delivery and minimizing radiation exposure to critical structures. The selection of these techniques depends on individual patient factors, tumor characteristics, and the availability of specialized treatment facilities. Collaborative decision-making between radiation oncologists, dermatologists, and other healthcare providers is crucial in determining the most suitable treatment approach for BCC patients.

## 8. Efficacy of radiation therapy for basal cell skin cancer

One of the primary goals of radiation therapy for basal cell carcinoma (BCC) is to achieve effective tumor control. Tumor control rates refer to the percentage of patients who experience local tumor control following radiation therapy. Several factors can influence tumor control rates, including tumor characteristics, treatment techniques, dose fractionation, and patient-specific factors. It is important to note that tumor control rates may vary depending on the specific studies and patient populations. Radiation therapy has demonstrated high rates of local control for primary BCCs. Studies have reported tumor control rates ranging from 90% to over 95% for primary tumors treated with radiation therapy alone. Tumor size, location, histological subtype, and depth of invasion can impact tumor control rates. Smaller, superficial tumors generally have higher control rates than more extensive, invasive tumors. The control rates for recurrent BCCs treated with radiation therapy can be more variable compared to primary tumors. They may range from 60–90%, depending on various factors, including the extent of recurrence, previous treatment history, and tumor biology. Radiation therapy can be an effective salvage treatment for recurrent BCCs, especially when surgical resection is challenging or not feasible due to anatomical constraints or patient comorbidities. Adjuvant radiation therapy may be recommended after surgical excision of high-risk BCCs to improve local control rates. The addition of radiation therapy to surgery has shown improved tumor control compared to surgery alone. Neoadjuvant radiation therapy refers to the administration of radiation therapy before surgery. It may be considered for large, locally advanced BCCs to downsize the tumor and facilitate surgical resection [20, 21].

Patient characteristics, including age, overall health status, and individual tumor factors, can influence tumor control rates. Patients with better overall health and favorable tumor characteristics tend to have higher tumor control rates. Patient compliance with the recommended treatment schedule and regular follow-up visits is essential for monitoring treatment response and detecting potential recurrence or late effects.

It is important to note that individual patient outcomes may vary, and treatment decisions should be made on a case-by-case basis, considering the patient's specific circumstances and the expertise of the multidisciplinary treatment team. Long-term follow-up and continued surveillance are essential to monitor tumor control and evaluate treatment success in BCC patients undergoing radiation therapy.

Cosmesis refers to the cosmetic appearance of the treated area following radiation therapy for basal cell carcinoma (BCC). Achieving favorable cosmesis outcomes is essential in managing BCC, as it contributes to the patient's overall quality of life and satisfaction with treatment. Several factors can influence cosmesis outcomes, including treatment techniques, dose fractionation, tumor characteristics, and individual patient factors. The use of advanced treatment techniques, such as 3D conformal radiation therapy (3D-CRT), intensity-modulated radiation therapy (IMRT), or volumetric modulated arc therapy (VMAT), can help in achieving better cosmesis outcomes. These techniques allow for more precise and conformal dose delivery, sparing healthy tissues and minimizing the impact on cosmetic appearance. Brachytherapy techniques, including surface brachytherapy and interstitial brachytherapy, can be advantageous in preserving cosmesis for superficial BCCs. These techniques provide targeted radiation delivery, minimizing damage to surrounding healthy tissues. The choice of dose fractionation schedule can impact cosmesis outcomes. Using standard fractionation schedules, such as delivering a total dose of 60–70 Gray (Gy) in daily fractions of 2 Gy over several weeks, has shown favorable cosmesis results. Hypofractionated regimens may also be considered, but long-term cosmesis outcomes are still being studied.

The location of the BCC can influence cosmesis outcomes. Tumors in cosmetically sensitive areas, such as the face, may require special attention to minimize cosmetic changes and ensure favorable outcomes. More extensive and deeper tumors may have a higher risk of affecting cosmesis due to the potential involvement of surrounding structures and the need for a more extensive treatment field. Tumor characteristics should be considered in treatment planning to optimize cosmesis outcomes. Discussing and understanding the patient's expectations regarding cosmesis outcomes is crucial. Managing realistic expectations and providing appropriate information about potential cosmetic changes can help ensure patient satisfaction. Individual patient factors, such as skin type and healing capacity, can affect cosmesis outcomes. Patients with sensitive or fragile skin may require special care and attention during treatment planning and delivery. Cosmesis outcomes should be evaluated immediately after treatment and during long-term follow-up visits. Regular assessment of cosmesis helps monitor the changes over time and address any concerns that may arise.

It is important to note that achieving optimal cosmesis outcomes in radiation therapy for BCC requires a multidisciplinary approach involving radiation oncologists, dermatologists, and other healthcare professionals. Collaboration and communication among the treatment team are essential to customize the treatment plan according to the patient's needs and optimize cosmesis results.

Long-term follow-up data plays a crucial role in evaluating the outcomes and assessing the efficacy of radiation therapy for basal cell carcinoma (BCC). It provides valuable information on tumor control rates, cosmesis outcomes, late effects, and overall treatment success. Long-term follow-up data allows for assessing local tumor control rates following radiation therapy. It provides information on the percentage of patients who remain free from local recurrence or progression of the treated BCC over an extended period. Long-term data helps determine the durability of tumor control achieved through radiation therapy. It allows for evaluating treatment effectiveness in preventing local recurrence over several years or even decades.

Long-term follow-up data includes cosmetic assessments of the treated area, providing information on the cosmetic appearance of the site after radiation therapy. It allows for evaluating cosmetic changes, such as skin pigmentation, texture, fibrosis, or other long-term effects on cosmesis. Long-term follow-up data may also include patient-reported outcomes regarding cosmesis and overall satisfaction with the cosmetic results. Patient feedback on their perceived cosmesis can provide valuable insights into the impact of radiation therapy on their quality of life.

Long-term follow-up data allows for assessing the late effects and potential treatment-related toxicities associated with radiation therapy for BCC. This includes evaluating the occurrence and severity of long-term skin changes, fibrosis, radiation dermatitis, or other late effects in the treated area. Long-term data also provide insights into the impact of radiation therapy on the patient's overall quality of life. This includes assessing functional outcomes, psychosocial well-being, and the impact of any late effects on daily activities or body image.

Long-term follow-up data enables the evaluation of disease-specific survival rates for BCC patients treated with radiation therapy. It provides information on the percentage of patients who survive without disease progression or metastasis. Long-term survival outcomes, including overall survival rates, can be assessed to determine the effectiveness of radiation therapy in improving long-term survival in BCC patients. Long-term follow-up data allows for comparative effectiveness studies, comparing radiation therapy outcomes with other treatment modalities, such as surgery or topical therapies. These studies help assess the long-term efficacy and advantages of radiation therapy in managing BCC. Pooling long-term follow-up data from multiple studies through meta-analyses provides a comprehensive evaluation of treatment outcomes and can strengthen the evidence base for radiation therapy in BCC.

Long-term follow-up data is crucial in monitoring treatment outcomes, understanding the long-term effects of radiation therapy, and informing clinical decision-making. It provides valuable insights into the efficacy, cosmesis outcomes, late effects, and overall survival rates associated with radiation therapy for BCC. Continual assessment and reporting of long-term follow-up data improve treatment strategies and patient care in the long run.

## 9. Adjuvant radiation therapy and combination approaches

Adjuvant radiation therapy refers to administering radiation treatment following primary surgical excision of basal cell carcinoma (BCC). It reduces the risk of local recurrence and improves treatment outcomes. Adjuvant radiation therapy is typically considered in cases with high-risk features, such as extensive tumor involvement, close or positive surgical margins, perineural invasion, or aggressive histological subtypes.

Adjuvant radiation therapy significantly reduces the risk of local recurrence in high-risk BCC cases. It targets residual microscopic disease in the surgical bed, enhancing local control rates. Adjuvant radiation therapy can spare patients from undergoing more extensive surgical procedures, especially in cases where surgical re-excision or reconstructive surgery poses significant morbidity. Adjuvant radiation therapy can help preserve organ function and achieve favorable cosmesis outcomes by avoiding extensive tissue removal during surgery [22, 23].

The presence of high-risk features, as determined by pathological evaluation of the excised tumor, is critical in determining the need for adjuvant radiation therapy. Radiation therapy planning for adjuvant treatment involves precise delineation of the surgical bed and surrounding areas at risk of microscopic disease. The treatment volume and dose are tailored to the individual patient's characteristics.

Combination approaches involve using multiple treatment modalities, such as surgery, radiation therapy, and systemic therapies, to optimize treatment outcomes in basal cell carcinoma. These approaches may be considered in cases with aggressive or advanced disease, where a multimodal approach is necessary to achieve local control and manage systemic spread.

In some instances, surgical excision followed by adjuvant radiation therapy may be employed to maximize local control rates and minimize the risk of recurrence. The combination of radiation therapy and systemic therapies, such as targeted therapies or immunotherapies, is an area of ongoing research. These combinations enhance treatment efficacy and improve outcomes, particularly in advanced or metastatic BCC cases.

Combination approaches require close collaboration between specialties, including surgical oncology, radiation oncology, medical oncology, and dermatology. A coordinated treatment plan ensures optimal sequencing and integration of therapies. The selection of patients for combination approaches depends on various factors, including disease stage, tumor characteristics, patient comorbidities, and treatment goals. Individualized treatment decisions are made based on a comprehensive patient condition evaluation.

Combination approaches, including adjuvant radiation therapy and multimodal therapies, offer potential benefits in managing basal cell carcinoma, particularly in cases with high-risk features or advanced disease. These approaches aim to improve local control rates, preserve function and cosmesis, and manage systemic disease. Adjuvant therapy and combination approaches should be tailored to each patient's needs, guided by multidisciplinary discussions and individualized treatment planning.

## 10. Side effects and toxicities of radiation therapy for basal cell skin cancer

Radiation therapy for basal cell carcinoma (BCC) can have acute and late effects on the skin and adjacent structures. These effects are important considerations in treatment planning and patient management [24]. Here, we discuss the potential acute and late effects associated with radiation therapy for BCC.

Acute Effects:

- Radiation Dermatitis: Acute radiation dermatitis is a common acute effect on the skin. It typically manifests as erythema (redness), dryness, and sometimes pruritus (itching). The severity of radiation dermatitis can vary depending on the dose, treatment technique, and individual patient factors. Proper skincare, topical agents, and patient education can help manage and minimize the impact of acute radiation dermatitis.

- Hair Loss: Depending on the treatment area, radiation therapy for BCC can result in temporary hair loss within the treatment field. This effect is typically reversible, and hair regrowth occurs several months after treatment completion.

- Fatigue: Radiation therapy can lead to fatigue, a common acute systemic effect. Patients may experience tiredness, lack of energy, and decreased ability to perform daily activities. Adequate rest, balanced nutrition, and regular physical activity can help manage treatment-related fatigue.

Late Effects:

- Radiation Fibrosis: Long-term radiation therapy can cause fibrosis in the treated area, leading to thickening and tightening of the skin. Fibrosis may cause functional limitations, particularly in areas with joint involvement. Physical therapy, regular movement, and skin moisturization can help mitigate the impact of radiation fibrosis.

- Telangiectasia: Telangiectasia is dilating small blood vessels near the skin's surface. It can result in red, spider-like veins on the skin. Telangiectasia is a potential late effect of radiation therapy and can persist long after treatment completion. Laser therapy or other interventions may be considered for management.

- Pigmentary Changes: Radiation therapy may cause pigmentary changes in the skin, including hypo- or hyperpigmentation. These changes can be permanent and affect the cosmetic appearance of the treated area. Sun protection measures, including sunscreen and protective clothing, are essential to minimize further pigmentation changes.

- Radiation-Induced Second Malignancies: Although rare, radiation therapy carries a small risk of inducing second malignancies, including skin cancers, in the treatment field. Regular surveillance and follow-up visits are crucial for detecting and managing potential secondary malignancies.

Effects on Adjacent Structures:

- Damage to Subcutaneous Tissues and Organs: Radiation therapy for BCC may affect subcutaneous tissues and nearby organs. The extent of damage depends on the treatment site and radiation dose. Potential effects include fibrosis, impaired wound healing, and functional impairment of adjacent structures.

- Bone and Cartilage Effects: In areas where bone or cartilage is exposed to radiation, long-term effects may include osteoradionecrosis (bone tissue death) or cartilage damage. These effects can lead to complications and require ongoing management and monitoring.

It is important to note that the severity and likelihood of acute and late effects can vary depending on various factors, including treatment technique, radiation dose, treatment volume, and individual patient characteristics. The multidisciplinary treatment team, including radiation oncologists, dermatologists, and supportive care professionals, plays a crucial role in assessing and managing these effects throughout the treatment process. Regular follow-up visits and long-term surveillance are essential to monitor and address any acute or late effects that may arise in patients undergoing radiation therapy for BCC.

Minimizing toxicities and optimizing patient comfort are essential goals in radiation therapy for basal cell carcinoma (BCC). Various strategies and interventions can be employed to reduce treatment-related toxicities and enhance the overall comfort of patients undergoing radiation therapy. Advanced treatment techniques, such as IMRT or VMAT, can help optimize dose distribution, sparing healthy tissues and reducing the risk of toxicities. IGRT techniques, such as daily imaging or real-time tracking, allow for accurate tumor targeting and minimize radiation exposure to surrounding healthy tissues, thus reducing potential toxicities. Careful treatment planning, including appropriate selection of beam angles, field arrangements, and dose constraints, helps minimize radiation exposure to critical structures, such as the eyes, salivary glands, or other organs at risk. Providing patients with comprehensive skincare education minimizes acute skin toxicities [25]. Patients should be instructed on proper skincare practices, such as gentle cleansing, moisturizing, and avoiding irritants or excessive sun exposure.

The use of approved topical agents, such as mild corticosteroids or emollients, may help alleviate acute radiation dermatitis and improve patient comfort. Emphasizing the importance of sun protection is essential to prevent further damage to the irradiated skin. Patients should be advised to use sunscreen, wear protective clothing, and limit sun exposure during and after treatment.

Adequate pain management is crucial to optimize patient comfort during and after radiation therapy. This may involve using analgesics, topical anesthetics, or other appropriate interventions tailored to the patient's needs. Maintaining proper nutrition is essential for patient comfort and recovery. Nutritional counseling or dietary interventions may be necessary to address treatment-related side effects, such as mucositis or dysphagia. Emotional support and counseling services can help alleviate anxiety or distress related to the diagnosis and treatment process. Support groups, individual therapy, or relaxation techniques may be beneficial in optimizing patient comfort.

Providing patients with detailed information about the treatment process, potential side effects, and self-care strategies empowers them to participate in their care and manage treatment-related toxicities actively. Involving patients in shared decision-making allows them to express their preferences and concerns [26]. This collaborative approach can help tailor treatment plans to individual needs, ensuring patient comfort and satisfaction. Regular follow-up visits and assessments allow for the early detection and management of treatment-related toxicities. Monitoring patients for acute and late effects ensures timely intervention and support. Implementing survivorship care plans that address the long-term needs of BCC survivors, including monitoring for potential late effects, supports optimal patient comfort and well-being in the posttreatment phase [27].

Minimizing toxicities and optimizing patient comfort requires a multidisciplinary approach involving radiation oncologists, dermatologists, nursing staff, and supportive care professionals. By employing comprehensive treatment planning strategies, providing appropriate supportive care measures, and fostering open communication with patients, radiation therapy for BCC can be delivered with a focus on minimizing toxicities and enhancing patient comfort.

## 11. Ongoing clinical trials and future perspectives

Ongoing clinical trials and future perspectives play a crucial role in advancing the field of radiation therapy for basal cell carcinoma (BCC) [28–33]. These endeavors aim to explore innovative treatment approaches, optimize treatment outcomes, and improve patient care. Clinical trials investigate combining radiation therapy with targeted therapies or immunotherapies in BCC treatment. These trials aim to determine the potential synergistic effects of combining radiation therapy with novel systemic agents, such as hedgehog pathways or immune checkpoint inhibitors.

Ongoing studies explore the use of radiosensitizing agents to enhance the effectiveness of radiation therapy in BCC. These agents may improve tumor response and reduce the required radiation dose, potentially minimizing toxicities while maximizing treatment outcomes. Clinical trials are evaluating shorter treatment schedules and hypofractionated radiation therapy regimens in BCC. These studies aim to assess the feasibility, efficacy, and potential benefits of delivering radiation therapy over a shorter period, reducing patient treatment burden. Ongoing studies investigate proton therapy, a form of external beam radiation therapy that delivers precise radiation doses to the tumor while minimizing radiation exposure to surrounding healthy tissues. Proton therapy may offer advantages in dose distribution and reduced toxicity in BCC treatment. Trials are exploring stereotactic radiation therapy, which delivers highly focused and precise radiation doses to the tumor while sparing nearby healthy tissues. These trials aim to assess the efficacy and safety of this technique in BCC treatment, particularly in cases where surgical intervention is challenging. Research efforts focus on developing predictive models and biomarkers to identify patients most likely to benefit from radiation therapy. These models may help guide treatment decision-making, optimize patient selection, and tailor treatment approaches based on individual patient characteristics.

The field of radiogenomics aims to identify genetic variations and radiographic features associated with treatment response and toxicities. Ongoing studies explore the potential of radiogenomics in predicting treatment outcomes and personalizing radiation therapy for BCC. Ongoing research emphasizes the importance of patient-reported outcomes, including quality-of-life assessments, symptom burden, and treatment-related toxicities. These studies aim to understand the impact of radiation therapy on patients' well-being and identify strategies to optimize patient comfort and satisfaction.

Future perspectives in radiation therapy for BCC also include advancements in treatment planning techniques, such as artificial intelligence-based algorithms for automated treatment planning and adaptive radiation therapy. These innovations may enhance treatment accuracy and efficiency and individualize treatment approaches further. It is important to note that clinical trials and ongoing research endeavors provide valuable insights and contribute to evidence-based practice. Patients and healthcare providers should stay informed about ongoing clinical trials and collaborate to ensure the incorporation of the latest scientific findings into clinical decision-making.

In conclusion, ongoing clinical trials and future perspectives in radiation therapy for BCC hold great promise in advancing treatment strategies, optimizing outcomes, and improving patient care. The exploration of targeted therapies, hypofractionation, advanced radiation techniques, predictive models, and patient-reported outcomes paves the way for personalized and patient-centered treatment approaches in the management of basal cell carcinoma. Continued research efforts and multidisciplinary collaborations are vital in shaping the future of radiation therapy for BCC and further improving patient outcomes and quality of life.

## Acknowledgements

We want to thank the people working at EVEX hospitals – Krystyna Kiel Oncology Center for their encouragement and advice that led to the completion of this paper.

We also thank our friends for their encouragement and words of advice. Special thanks to Krystyna Kiel. Finally, if not for our families, who support us always, we would never be able to work on this extraordinary project.

The author acknowledges the use of Grammarly for the language polishing of the manuscript.

## Conflict of interest

The author declared no potential conflicts of interest with respect to the research, authorship, and publication of this article. This research did not receive a specific grant from funding agencies in the public, commercial, or not-for-profit sectors.

## Acronyms and abbreviations

| | |
|---|---|
| BCC | basal cell carcinoma |
| RT | radiation therapy |
| EBRT | external beam radiation therapy |
| HDR | high-dose rate |
| NMSC | nonmelanoma skin cancer |
| CT | clinical trials |
| IMRT | intensity-modulated radiation therapy |
| OARs | organs at risk |
| PTV | planning target volume |
| AD | acute dermatitis |
| LENT/SOMA | late effects normal tissue/symptom occurrence and management analysis |
| EBD | electronic brachytherapy device |
| APBI | accelerated partial breast irradiation |
| PNI | perineural invasion |
| HNC | head and neck cancer |
| CTV | clinical target volume |
| SBRT | stereotactic body radiation therapy |
| VMAT | volumetric modulated arc therapy |
| PRD | proton radiation dermatitis |
| SIB | simultaneous integrated boost |
| NCCN | national comprehensive cancer network |
| SCC | squamous cell carcinoma |
| RTOG | radiation therapy oncology group |
| CTCAE | common terminology criteria for adverse events |
| RBE | relative biological effectiveness |
| EORTC | European organization for research and treatment of cancer |
| MOSF | margins of safety for critical structures |
| IMPT | intensity-modulated proton therapy |
| RPA | radiation planning assistant |
| ONS | oncology nursing society |
| AJCC | American joint committee on cancer |
| PS-SDRT | pulse-dose superficial radiation therapy |
| DFS | disease-free survival |

| | |
|---|---|
| OS | overall survival |
| LC | local control |
| RILD | radiation-induced liver disease |
| V20 | percentage of lung volume receiving 20 gy or more |
| V50 | percentage of lung volume receiving 50 gy or more |
| SRS | stereotactic radiosurgery |
| HU | hounsfield units |
| IORT | intraoperative radiation therapy |
| CI | confidence interval |
| QoL | quality of life |
| OAR | organ at risk |
| Dmax | maximum dose |
| D95 | dose received by 95% of the target volume |
| NTCP | normal tissue complication probability |
| BED | biologically effective dose |
| CR | complete response |
| PR | partial response |
| NR | no response |
| TNM | tumor, node, metastasis |
| LRC | locoregional control |
| DRR | digitally reconstructed radiograph |
| HDR-BT | high-dose-rate brachytherapy |
| CT-Sim | computed tomography simulation |
| GTV | gross tumor volume |
| OSLD | optically stimulated luminescent dosimeter |
| R&V | record and verify |

## Author details

Eter Natelauri[1*] and Anna Jghamadze[2]

1 EVEX Hospitals-Krystyna Kiel Oncology Center, Kutaisi, Georgia

2 VIAN - Krystyna Kiel Oncology Center, Kutaisi, Georgia

*Address all correspondence to: enatelauri@yahoo.com

## References

[1] Lomas A, Leonardi-Bee J, Bath-Hextall F. A systematic review of worldwide incidence of nonmelanoma skin cancer. The British Journal of Dermatology. 2012;**166**(5):1069-1080. DOI: 10.1111/j.1365-2133.2012.10830.x

[2] Leiter U, Keim U, Garbe C. Epidemiology of skin cancer: Update 2019. Advances in Experimental Medicine and Biology. 2020;**1268**:123-139. DOI: 10.1007/978-3-030-46227-7_6

[3] Smeets NW, Krekels GA, Ostertag JU, Essers BA, Dirksen CD, Nieman FH, et al. Surgical excision vs Mohs' micrographic surgery for basal-cell carcinoma of the face: Randomised controlled trial. Lancet (London, England). 2004;**364**(9447):1766-1772. DOI: 10.1016/S0140-6736(04)17399-6

[4] Rubin AI, Chen EH, Ratner D. Basal-cell carcinoma. The New England Journal of Medicine. 2005;**353**(21):2262-2269. DOI: 10.1056/NEJMra044151

[5] Cameron MC, Lee E, Hibler BP, Barker CA, Mori S, Cordova M, et al. Basal cell carcinoma: Epidemiology; pathophysiology; clinical and histological subtypes; and disease associations. Journal of the American Academy of Dermatology. 2019;**80**(2):303-317. DOI: 10.1016/j.jaad.2018.03.060

[6] Lallas A, Tzellos T, Kyrgidis A, Apalla Z, Zalaudek I, Karatolias A, et al. Accuracy of dermoscopic criteria for discriminating superficial from other subtypes of basal cell carcinoma. Journal of the American Academy of Dermatology. 2014;**70**(2):303-311. DOI: 10.1016/j.jaad.2013.10.003

[7] Peris K, Fargnoli MC, Garbe C, Kaufmann R, Bastholt L, Seguin NB, et al. Diagnosis and treatment of basal cell carcinoma: European consensus-based interdisciplinary guidelines. European Journal of Cancer (Oxford, England: 1990). 2019;**118**:10-34. DOI: 10.1016/j.ejca.2019.06.003

[8] National Comprehensive Cancer Network (NCCN). NCCN Clinical Practice Guidelines in Oncology (NCCN Guidelines®): Basal Cell Skin Cancer. Version 1.2023. PA: National Comprehensive Cancer Network (NCCN). Available from: https://www.nccn.org/professionals/physician_gls/pdf/nmsc.pdf; [Accessed: May 20, 2023]

[9] Cheraghi N, Cognetta A, Goldberg D. Radiation therapy in dermatology: Non-melanoma skin cancer. Journal of Drugs in Dermatology: JDD. 2017;**16**(5):464-469

[10] Ko HC, Gupta V, Mourad WF, Hu KS, Harrison LB, Som PM, et al. A contouring guide for head and neck cancers with perineural invasion. Practical Radiation Oncology. 2014;**4**(6):e247-e258. DOI: 10.1016/j.prro.2014.02.001

[11] Gunaratne DA, Veness MJ. Efficacy of hypofractionated radiotherapy in patients with non-melanoma skin cancer: Results of a systematic review. Journal of Medical Imaging and Radiation Oncology. 2018;**62**(3):401-411. DOI: 10.1111/1754-9485.12718

[12] Lliso F, Granero D, Perez-Calatayud J, Carmona V, Pujades MC, Ballester F. Dosimetric evaluation of internal shielding in a high dose rate skin applicator. Journal of Contemporary Brachytherapy. 2011;**3**(1):32-35. DOI: 10.5114/jcb.2011.21041

[13] Lasota J, Kabacińska R, Makarewicz R. Dose estimation for different skin models in interstitial breast brachytherapy. Journal of Contemporary Brachytherapy. 2014;**6**(2):200-207. DOI: 10.5114/jcb.2014.43167

[14] Nag S, Cano ER, Demanes DJ, Puthawala AA, Vikram B, American Brachytherapy Society. The American brachytherapy society recommendations for high-dose-rate brachytherapy for head-and-neck carcinoma. International Journal of Radiation Oncology, Biology, Physics. 2001;**50**(5):1190-1198. DOI: 10.1016/s0360-3016(01)01567-x

[15] Toller G, Lakosi F, Antal G, Kovacs A, Battyani Z, Repa I, et al. CT assisted 3D high-dose-rate brachytherapy (HDR-BT) in the treatment of skin carcinomas. Journal of Contemporary Brachytherapy. 2009;**1**(3):190-191

[16] Rio E, Bardet E, Ferron C, Peuvrel P, Supiot S, Campion L, et al. Interstitial brachytherapy of periorificial skin carcinomas of the face: A retrospective study of 97 cases. International Journal of Radiation Oncology, Biology, Physics. 2005;**63**(3):753-757. DOI: 10.1016/j.ijrobp.2005.03.027

[17] Wilder RB, Kittelson JM, Shimm DS. Basal cell carcinoma treated with radiation therapy. Cancer. 1991;**68**(10):2134-2137. DOI: 10.1002/1097-0142(19911115)68:10<2134::aid-cncr2820681008>3.0.co;2-m

[18] Skowronek J. Brachytherapy in the treatment of skin cancer: An overview. Postepy Dermatologii I Alergologii. 2015;**32**(5):362-367. DOI: 10.5114/pdia.2015.54746

[19] Umebayashi Y, Uyeno K, Tsujii H, Otsuka F. Proton radiotherapy of skin carcinomas. The British Journal of Dermatology. 1994;**130**(1):88-91. DOI: 10.1111/j.1365-2133.1994.tb06889.x

[20] Kurian RR, Di Palma S, Barrett AW. Basal cell carcinoma metastatic to parotid gland. Head and Neck Pathology. 2014;**8**(3):349-353. DOI: 10.1007/s12105-013-0507-3

[21] Mohan SV, Chang AL. Advanced basal cell carcinoma: Epidemiology and therapeutic innovations. Current Dermatology Reports. 2014;**3**(1):40-45. DOI: 10.1007/s13671-014-0069-y

[22] Avril MF, Auperin A, Margulis A, Gerbaulet A, Duvillard P, Benhamou E, Guillaume JC, Chalon R, Petit JY, Sancho-Garnier H, Prade M, Bouzy J, Chassagne D. Basal cell carcinoma of the face: Surgery or radiotherapy? Results of a randomized study. British Journal of Cancer. 1997;**76**(1):100-106. DOI: 10.1038/bjc.1997.343

[23] Likhacheva A, Awan M, Barker CA, Bhatnagar A, Bradfield L, Brady MS, et al. Definitive and postoperative radiation therapy for basal and squamous cell cancers of the skin: Executive summary of an American Society for Radiation Oncology clinical practice guideline. Practical Radiation Oncology. 2020;**10**(1):8-20. DOI: 10.1016/j.prro.2019.10.014

[24] Russi EG, Moretto F, Rampino M, Benasso M, Bacigalupo A, De Sanctis V, et al. Acute skin toxicity management in head and neck cancer patients treated with radiotherapy and chemotherapy or EGFR inhibitors: Literature review and consensus. Critical Reviews in Oncology/Hematology. 2015;**96**(1):167-182. DOI: 10.1016/j.critrevonc.2015.06.001

[25] Bensadoun RJ, Humbert P, Krutman J, Luger T, Triller R, Rougier A, et al. Daily baseline skin care in the prevention, treatment, and supportive

care of skin toxicity in oncology patients: Recommendations from a multinational expert panel. Cancer Management and Research. 2013;**5**:401-408. DOI: 10.2147/CMAR.S52256

[26] Elwyn G, Frosch D, Thomson R, Joseph-Williams N, Lloyd A, Kinnersley P, et al. Shared decision making: A model for clinical practice. Journal of General Internal Medicine. 2012;**27**(10):1361-1367. DOI: 10.1007/s11606-012-2077-6. Epub 2012 May 23

[27] Pergolotti M, Deal AM, Williams GR, Bryant AL, Bensen JT, Muss HB, et al. Activities, function, and health-related quality of life (HRQOL) of older adults with cancer. Journal of Geriatric Oncology. 2017;**8**(4):249-254. DOI: 10.1016/j.jgo.2017.02.009

[28] Stratigos AJ, Sekulic A, Peris K, Bechter O, Prey S, Kaatz M, et al. Cemiplimab in locally advanced basal cell carcinoma after hedgehog inhibitor therapy: An open-label, multi-Centre, single-arm, phase 2 trial. The Lancet. Oncology. 2021;**22**(6):848-857. DOI: 10.1016/S1470-2045(21)00126-1

[29] Basset-Seguin N, Hauschild A, Grob JJ, Kunstfeld R, Dréno B, Mortier L, et al. Vismodegib in patients with advanced basal cell carcinoma (STEVIE): A pre-planned interim analysis of an international, open-label trial. The Lancet. Oncology. 2015;**16**(6):729-736. DOI: 10.1016/S1470-2045(15)70198-1

[30] Chapman CH, Nookala P, Bernardo SG, et al. Safety and efficacy of proton beam therapy for advanced hepatocellular carcinoma: Results of a phase I trial. International Journal of Radiation Oncology, Biology, Physics. 2020;**108**(5):1202-1211. DOI: 10.1016/j.ijrobp.2020.07.020

[31] West CM, Barnett GC. Genetics and genomics of radiotherapy toxicity: Towards prediction. Genome Medicine. 2011;**3**(8):52. DOI: 10.1186/gm268

[32] Jackson L, Larson G, Deshmukh S, et al. Radiogenomics of head and neck squamous cell carcinoma: Machine learning-based pretreatment computed tomography texture and radiomics classifiers to predict locoregional failure and survival outcomes. International Journal of Radiation Oncology, Biology, Physics. 2020;**108**(1):238-245. DOI: 10.1016/j.ijrobp.2020.02.031

[33] Ng J, Dai T. Radiation therapy and the abscopal effect: A concept comes of age. Annals of Translational Medicine. 2016;**4**(6):118. DOI: 10.21037/atm.2016.01.32

Chapter 6

# Topical Fluorouracil Therapy for Basal Cell Carcinoma

*Csongor Németh, Rolland Gyulai and Zsuzsanna Lengyel*

## Abstract

Basal cell carcinoma is a nonmelanoma skin cancer and is the commonest malignancy of the skin. It accounts for approximately 80% of all skin cancers and is encountered frequently in daily clinical practice. The nonsurgical methods in the treatment of basal cell carcinoma gain more and more attention due to the increasing incidence of the tumor and the aging population. The authors hereby summarize the therapeutic place of topical 5-fluorouracil in the treatment of basal cell carcinoma. They review the mechanism, effectiveness of the therapeutic agent, how it should be applied by the patient, and the possible side effects. The chapter is also illustrated with cases.

**Keywords:** topical therapy, fluorouracil, basal cell carcinoma

## 1. Introduction

Basal cell carcinoma (BCC) accounts for 80% of all nonmelanoma skin cancers and is the most common malignant tumor in the Caucasian population [1]. The treatment of basal cell carcinoma depends on the tumor, the individual risk factors (like age, comorbidities, performance status, and preference), the available treatment options, and the preference or expertise of the treating clinician/physician.

The goal of treatment is the complete removal of the tumor with the least cosmetic and functional impact [2]. Treatment modalities can be divided into surgical and nonsurgical methods. Surgical treatments are standard excision, microscopically controlled surgery or Mohs micrographic surgery, curettage, electrodessication, cryosurgery, and laser therapy. Nonsurgical therapies include topical treatments (5-fluorouracil, imiquimod), radiotherapy, photodynamic therapy, electrochemotherapy, and systemic therapy (vismodegib, sonidegib, cemiplimab, pembrolizumab). Several factors influence the choice of which treatment will be sufficient. A new classification proposed by European consensus-based interdisciplinary guidance divides the tumors into two groups based on their difficulty to treat ("easy-to-treat" (common) BCC vs. "difficult-to-treat" BCC). The first line treatment of BCCs, according to the international guidelines, is the complete surgical excision with histological confirmation of the subtype and margins of the tumor.

Microscopically controlled surgery should be chosen for high-risk BCC, recurrent BCC, and BCC in critical anatomical sites [3]. If the clinical-dermoscopic examination shows features of superficial BCC (sBCC) without any high-risk BCC features, then topical therapies and other destructive therapies can be considered, though the cure rate is lower than with surgical treatment.

Another important consideration of treatment choice is the risk of recurrence. sBCCs treated with nonsurgical methods show a higher risk of recurrence compared to surgical treatment with available histopathology.

Also, when choosing a nonsurgical method, the localization of sBCC should be taken into consideration as the recurrence of the tumor on the back has a better prognosis and is easier to manage than a recurrence of a high-risk BCC on the face [2, 3].

When deciding whether to treat a superficial basal cell carcinoma surgically or nonsurgically, our therapeutic decision is influenced by several factors of the patient such as age, comorbidities, medications, and social circumstances. Older people often refuse surgical interventions due to the inconvenience.

## 2. Superficial basal cell carcinoma clinical and dermoscopic features

Superficial BCC is the second most common clinical subtype, accounting for up to 15% of cases [4]. Superficial BCCs appear most commonly on the trunk and extremities, in contrast to the other subtypes, which favor head and neck localization. The mean age at diagnosis is 57 years, suggesting that this subtype occurs at a younger age compared to other subtypes [5]. sBCC typically appears as a well-circumscribed, scaly, pink-to-red macule, patch, thin papule, or thin plaque. It may show as a crust or a thin rolled border consisting of fine translucent small papules. Areas of spontaneous regression can occur, leaving behind atrophic, hypopigmented areas. Variable amounts of melanin pigment may be present [6].

Dermoscopic features of superficial basalioma are short-fine vessels, multiple small erosions, and shiny white structures. In addition, 79% of lesions present with the shiny white-red structureless background. When pigmentation is present, it most commonly appears as multiple brown dots and globules, spoke wheel, and leaf-like areas [7].

## 3. Topical therapies in the management of superficial basal cell carcinomas

The two most common topical treatments in the management of basal cell carcinoma are imiquimod and 5-fluorouracil-containing cream, and the combination of these therapies with other modalities.

Nowadays, other novel topical therapies are under investigation, for example, topical hedgehog pathway inhibitors (HPI) (sonidegib, patidegib) and histone deacetylase (HDAC) inhibitors (vorinostat, remetinostat). They are targeting the molecular inhibition of aberrantly overactivated hedgehog signaling. A phase II study of sporadic nodular BCC and superficial BCC treated with topical sonidegib was terminated early due to a lack of efficacy [8]. A phase I study for a novel topical HPI, CUR61414, also did not show efficacy [9]. Patidegib 2% or 4% gel was being evaluated in several clinical trials for patients with basal cell nevoid syndrome (BCNS, Gorlin-Goltz Syndrome) and in non-syndromic patients with high-frequency BCCs (NCT02762084, NCT02828111). The results of both trials demonstrated that patidegib 2% gel has a higher clinical (reduction of 51.29% in the number of tumors) and molecular (reduction of –56.3% in the GLI1mRNA levels) efficacy on BCC, with less

AEs, than the 4% gel [10]. Remetinostat 1% gel applied three times daily for 6 weeks, was evaluated in phase II open trial of 25 patients with 33 BCCs. The pathological resolution was seen in 54.8% of tumors, but response varied by histological subtype with 100% of sBCCs, 68.2% of nBCCs, and 66.7% of iBCCs responding. No serious adverse events were reported. The most common side effect was treatment site dermatitis [11]. Topical HPIs and HDAC inhibitors are still being investigated even though they are not yet clinically available [12].

Imiquimod is an immunomodulator drug used topically against cutaneous viral infections and tumors. The United States Food and Drug Administration approved imiquimod under the brand name Aldara in 1997 for the treatment of genital and perianal warts, and the treatment of typical, nonhyperkeratotic, and nonhypertrophic actinic keratoses on the face or scalp in immunocompetent adults. The FDA approved imiquimod for the topical treatment of sBCC in 2004, specifically biopsy-proven primary sBCC in immunocompetent adults with largest diameter of 2.0 cm, located on the trunk (barring anogenital region), neck, or extremities (excluding hands and feet) in immunocompetent adults when surgical methods are not available or inappropriate [13, 14]. Imiquimod acts through the toll-like receptor (TLR) 7 and 8. It activates both the innate and the adaptive immune systems and enhances the production of cytokines and natural killer cells, the proliferation of B lymphocytes, and the activation of Langerhans cells. This treatment causes inflammation at the tumor site, due to stimulation of the immune response, resulting in erythema, edema, scaling, and erosions. In a prospective trial, superficial BCCs treated with imiquimod cream 5% once daily seven times per week for 6 weeks showed a 5-year cure rate of 85% [15]. In a phase III randomized controlled trial treating superficial BCC and nodular BCC with 5% imiquimod applied once daily 5 days a week for 6 weeks showed an 84% cure rate at 3 years [16].

### 3.1 Fluorouracil

5-fluorouracil (5-FU) is an antimetabolite that impairs DNA replication by blocking the synthesis of thymidylate. Systemic use of 5-FU is FDA/EMA-indicated for treating gastric adenocarcinoma, pancreatic adenocarcinoma, breast carcinoma, and colorectal adenocarcinoma. Topical 5-FU is commonly used as a first-line treatment for malignant and premalignant skin conditions [17]. 5-FU first appeared in 1957 as a new chemotherapeutic drug. In the early 1960s, topical use of 5-FU showed cytotoxic effects in some skin cancers and precursor lesions. In 1970, FDA approved 5-FU (in 1% and 5% formulations) for topical use [18]. The indication for therapy by 5-FU is the nonmelanoma skin cancers and their precursor lesions. We have good evidence-based data in the treatment of actinic keratosis, especially in the field treatment [19], but the evidence in the treatment of keratoacanthomas and squamous cell carcinoma *in situ* is limited [20]. Later in this chapter, the studies with 5-FU in the treatment of sBCCs will be mentioned.

#### *3.1.1 5-Fluorouracil mechanism of action*

As mentioned earlier, 5-fluorouracil belongs to the antimetabolite chemotherapeutic drugs. 5-FU is a heterocyclic aromatic organic compound with a structure similar to that of the pyrimidine molecules of DNA and RNA; it is an analog of uracil with a fluorine atom at the C-5 position in place of hydrogen [18]. It has three main methods of action:

1. 5-FU is a thymidylate synthase inhibitor. Thymidylate synthase (TS) catalyzes the methylation of deoxyuridine monophosphate (dUMP) to deoxythimidine monophosphate (dTMP). 5-FU is transported into the cell, where 5-FU is converted to fluorodeoxyuridine monophosphate (FdUMP), fluorodeoxyuridine triphosphate (FdUTP), and fluorouridine triphosphate (FUTP). The normal synthesis and functioning of DNA and RNA are affected by these abnormal metabolites by forming a stable complex with thymidylate synthase, leading to the inhibition of deoxythymidine monophosphate (dTMP) production. The cytotoxicity is due to the impairment of DNA replication and repair because of the depletion of dTMP, so the rapidly dividing tumor cells undergo death owing to the lack of dTMP [21].

2. 5-FU is a pyrimidine analog that can be misincorporated into RNA and DNA in place of uracil or thymine. The abnormal 5-FU antimetabolites are misincorporated into DNA, which demands excision and repair of DNA. The increased requirement of DNA repair leads to DNA strand breaks and ultimately cell death in mammalian cells [22]. 5-FU can also be misincorporated into RNA and interfere with many aspects of RNA function, inhibiting the processing of pre-rRNA into mature rRNA, modification of tRNAs, and the inhibition of the splicing of pre-mRNA [23].

3. Another hypothesized mechanism of action is the interference with p53. p53 induce cell-cycle arrest and apoptosis in cells with DNA damage. Topical administration of 5-FU may result in stimulation of p53-mediated apoptosis of the rapidly proliferating cells found in dermatological lesions with altered p53 expression like sBCC, actinic keratosis, and squamous cell carcinoma [24]. In a study gene and protein expression of various molecules were measured after topical fluorouracil treatment. They observed an increase in keratin 16, interleukin-1b, matrix metalloproteinase-1 and -3 mRNA levels. These latter molecules are also increased in the wound healing process, suggesting that after damage fluorouracil may be inducing a healing response as well [18, 25].

### *3.1.2 Topical formulations*

In the case of topical application cytotoxicity with 5-FU occurs only in the rapidly proliferating cells of abnormal skin, leaving normal skin cell types relatively unaffected. A hypothetical method of action of topical 5-FU is the inhibition of TS activity completely in actinic/injured skin [20].

5-FU is available in the following forms: 0.5%, 1%, 2%, 4%, and 5% cream and there is a combination of 0.5% 5-FU + 10% salicylic acid.

In Europe, topical 5-fluorouracil is currently marketed in two different concentrations 0.5% and 5%. The 0.5% solution contains 10% salicylic acid and is indicated for the topical treatment of slightly palpable and/or moderately thick hyperkeratotic actinic keratosis in immunocompetent adult patients, as well as to treat warts. The 5% cream formula (Efudix®) is indicated for the topical treatment of superficial premalignant and malignant skin lesions; keratoses, including senile, actinic and arsenical forms, keratoacanthoma, Bowen's disease, and superficial BCC [26].

In the USA, Efudex® Solution contains 2% or 5% fluorouracil. Efudex® cream contains 5% fluorouracil. They are approved for the treatment of actinic keratosis (AK) using the 5% fluorouracil cream in the treatment of sBCCs. The other available

5-FU-containing creams are administered in AK treatment, for example, Fluoroplex® 1% topical cream twice daily, for a treatment period of 2–6 weeks, Tolak® 4% cream once each day for 4 weeks, and Carac ® cream once daily for 4 weeks.

Among these preparations, only 5% 5-FU cream is registered to treat sBCCs [19].

### *3.1.3 Studies on efficacy of 5-FU in the treatment of superficial BCC*

Topical 5-FU has been used in the treatment of basal cell carcinoma since the 1960s. In the early studies, the concentration of 5-FU varied between 1 and 30%, the application length was approximately 6 weeks or more. The reported clearance rate was 56–80% and only one study claimed 90% in which the concentration of 5-FU was 30% [27–30]. The higher concentration was linked to more frequent and severe side effects. In 1970, 5% 5-FU was the first topical therapy approved by the U.S. Food and Drug Administration for the treatment of superficial BCCs. This approval was based on a study of 113 superficial BCC lesions in 54 patients, which demonstrated a 93% complete clearance rate [31]. The recommended mode of application is twice daily, at least for 3–6 weeks. Since then, few clinical trials have been conducted with 5-FU cream for sBCCs.

In 2007, a clinical study was performed where the authors evaluated, with a histologic endpoint, the efficacy, tolerability, cosmetic outcome, and patient satisfaction of 5% 5-FU therapy in superficial BCC. The 5-FU cream was applied twice daily for up to 12 weeks. The treated lesion was excised and histologically examined 3 weeks after the end of treatment. The histologic cure rate was 90% and the therapy was well tolerated with good cosmetic outcomes [32].

In a single-blinded, randomized controlled multicenter trial, conducted in Netherlands, patients were assigned for treatment with methyl aminolevulinate-photodynamic therapy (MAL-PDT, two sessions with an interval of 1 week), imiquimod cream (once daily, five times a week for 6 weeks), or fluorouracil cream (twice daily for 4 weeks). 601 patients were enrolled in the study. The proportion of patients, tumor-free at both 3- and 12-month follow-up was 72.8% (95% CI 66.8–79.4) for MAL-PDT, 83.4% (78.2–88.9) for imiquimod cream, and 80.1% (74.7–85.9) for fluorouracil cream. The authors concluded that topical fluorouracil was non-inferior and imiquimod was superior to MAL-PDT for the treatment of superficial basal-cell carcinoma [33].

The 5-year follow-up results of this study were presented in 2018. The authors found that the probability of tumor-free survival was 62.7% for MAL-PDT therapy (95% confidence interval [CI] = 55.3–69.2), 80.5% for imiquimod (95% CI = 74.0–85.6), and 70.0% for 5-fluorouracil (95% CI = 62.9–76.0) after 5 years of treatment. The hazard ratio for treatment failure of imiquimod and 5-fluorouracil were 0.48 (95% CI = 0.32–0.71, $P < 0.001$) and 0.74 (95% CI = 0.53–1.05, $P = 0.09$), respectively, when compared with MAL-PDT therapy. Compared with 5-fluorouracil, imiquimod showed a hazard ratio of 0.65 (95% CI 0.43–0.98, $P = 0.04$). In summary, 5 years after treatment, 5% imiquimod cream was proven to be superior to both MAL-PDT and topical 5-FU cream. Based on these findings, the authors recommend the use of 5% imiquimod cream as the first choice for noninvasive treatment in most primary superficial basal cell carcinomas [34].

In a recent retrospective study, 350 patients with sBCC and 411 *in situ* squamous cell carcinoma were enrolled. In the treatment of epidermal carcinomas surgical, destructive therapy or topical 5% FU was used. In a comparison of all methods, treatment with 5-FU had the most failures (12.5%) for sBCC, although compared with the failure rates of surgical (3.7%) and destructive (5.2%) modalities, differences did not reach statistical significance. Regarding this real-world data, the outcomes of topical 5-FU for both SCCIS and sBCC showed an overall success rate of greater than 90% (92.9% for SCCIS and 87.5% for sBCC) in a cohort with a mean clearance follow-up of 41 months. The authors concluded that 5-FU is an appropriate nonsurgical method for sBCC, although lesion and patient factors must be considered [35].

#### *3.1.4 Combination therapies with 5-fluorouracil*

By altering the skin barrier, there is a possibility to enhance the penetration of the chemotherapeutic drug. Different chemicals and physical tools can increase the efficacy of 5-FU like occlusion [36], microemulsions and liposomes [37, 38], microneedles [39], iontophoresis, electroporation [40], laser-assisted drug delivery [41, 42], salicylic acid, and cryotherapy [43].

In a case study series with two patients, 0.5% 5-fluorouracil and 10% salicylic acid (5-FU-SA) were used once a day at night for 6 weeks for multiple pigmented sBCCs. After 6 weeks of application, clinical and dermoscopical examination confirmed complete regression of the lesions, which was also confirmed by the histopathological findings. No recurrences were seen at 6 months of follow-up. The authors attributed the good result to the better penetration of 5-FU induced by the keratolytic effect of salicylic acid [44].

In a study, ablative fractional laser (AFL) was used followed by a single application of topical 5% 5-FU under occlusion for 7 days for 30 primary sBCC and SCCis lesions, measured less than 2 cm on the trunk and extremities. Histologic clearance was 87% overall, 100% (16/16) for SCCis vs. 71% for sBCC [41].

In another follow-up study, ablative fractional laser (AFL) assisted delivery of cisplatin and 5-FU in low-risk BCCs showed complete tumor clearance of 89% and 79% at 6 and 12 months, respectively. The clearance rate for sBCCs 1 year after treatment was 100% and lower for nodular BCC at 69% [42].

In a study by Soong et al., sBCCs and SCCis were treated with cryotherapy (liquid nitrogen, 10 s, 2 mm margins, distance of 1–2 cm). After a 1-month healing period patients completed a 3-week course of 5% 5-FU applied twice daily. Among the sBCCs, 30 lesions of the 34 that were assessed, demonstrated no evidence of recurrence at a mean follow-up time of 6.6 months [43].

#### *3.1.5 Systemic absorption of topical 5-FU*

The commercially available formulations show poor skin permeation and retention of 5-FU and cytotoxicity occurs only in the rapidly proliferating cells of abnormal skin.

Dillaha et al. found that the cutaneous absorption rate after topical application of 5-FU was approximately 6% in their study, a too small amount to cause systemic side effects [45]. According to the Efudix package insert, application on skin areas over 529 $cm^2$ (23 × 23 cm) is not recommended [46]. In affected skin, the rate of absorption was raised to about 15–75 times that of healthy skin but this quantity of 5-FU in a large area like 200 $cm^2$, could still be considered as unable to induce systemic toxicity [47]. In a comparison of the pharmacokinetics of 0.5% fluorouracil and 5% fluorouracil in actinic keratosis, it was found that the drug plasma concentration was detectable 60% more often in the 5% FU group and the cumulative amount excreted in the urine of the 0.5% fluorouracil group was approximately one-fortieth that of the 5% fluorouracil group. The side effects were less in the 0.5% group [48]. New drug formulations like nanostructured lipid carrier-based hydrogels can enhance the 5-FU penetration potential into the epidermis and dermis layers in *in vivo* studies and can possibly reduce systemic access and side effects compared to 5-FU conventional formulations such as cream, gel, and ointment [49]. Dihydropyrimidine dehydrogenase (DPD) is a key enzyme involved in metabolizing and eliminating fluorouracil. Systemic drug toxicity

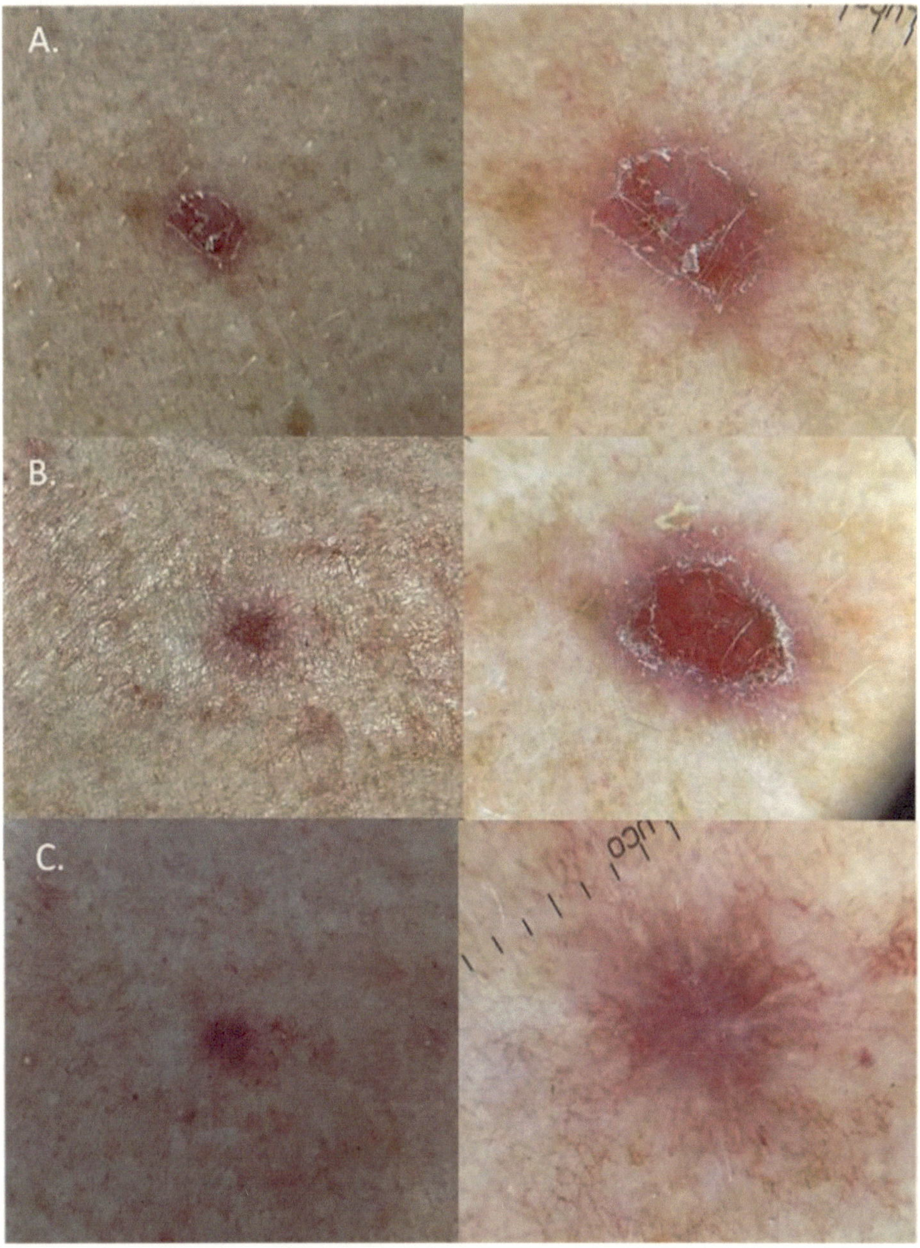


**Figure 1.**
*45-year-old female patient with multiple sBCCs treated with 5% 5FU cream. Lesion located on the chest clinical and dermoscopy picture (A). At 2 weeks of treatment, moderate inflammation and ulceration are depicted in the photos (B). Two weeks after cessation of therapy, complete healing of the lesion and no sign of malignancy on the dermoscopic image (C).*

is increased in patients who have reduced activity of DPD, because they are unable to convert 5-FU to a biologically inactive metabolite. In these cases, DPD activity determination has to be considered, but the incidence of this is very low [50].

### *3.1.6 Side effects of topical 5-FU*

Normal skin reactions to the treatment are redness, dryness, tenderness, and later crusts appear with erosions and minimal bleeding (**Figures 1** and **2**). The clinical manifestation of response usually occurs in the second week of 5-FU treatment.

The most common side effects from topical 5-FU include irritant dermatitis with associated erythema, dryness, pain, burning, and itching (**Figures 3** and **4**). Other

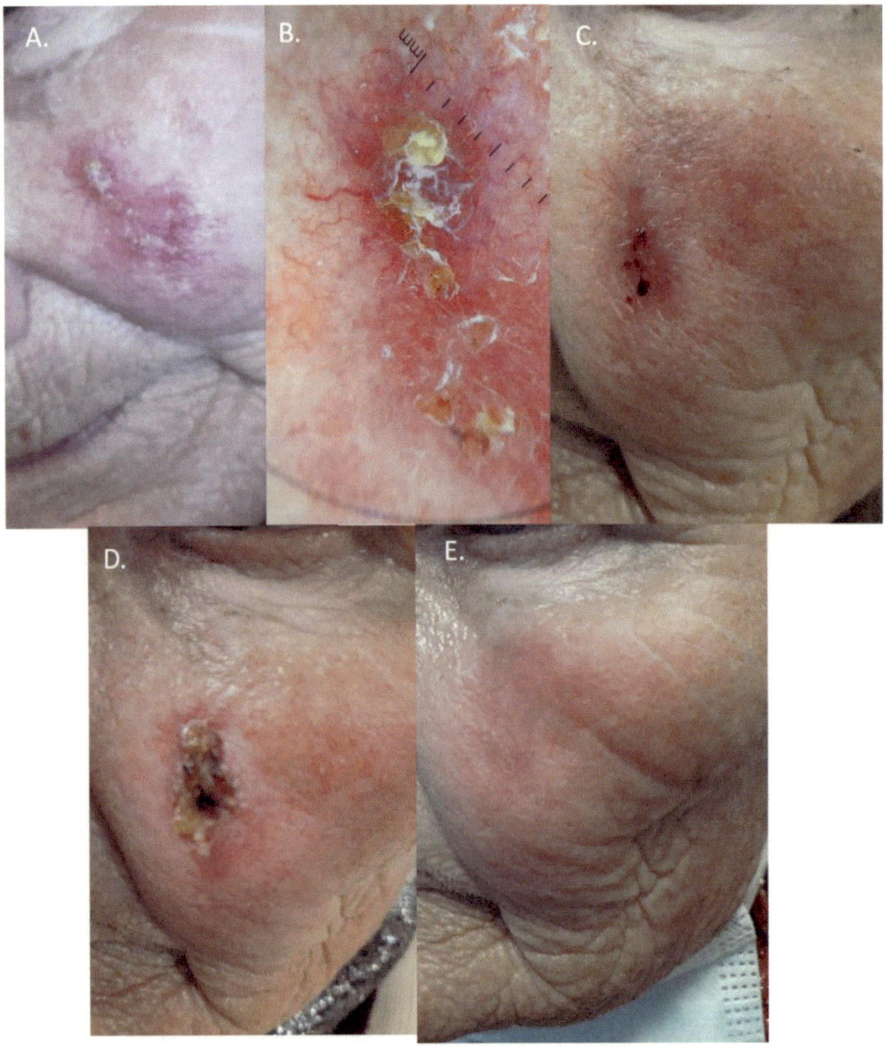


**Figure 2.**
*89-year-old female patient with basal cell carcinoma on the left cheek. The lower part of the lesion was more infiltrative (A). Linear vessels and multiple erosions were seen with dermoscopy (B). Two weeks after the initiation of 5% 5-FU cream inflammation was already seen (C). Later, oozing and crusting occurred (D). Three weeks after cessation of 5-FU treatment, complete regression of BCC (E).*

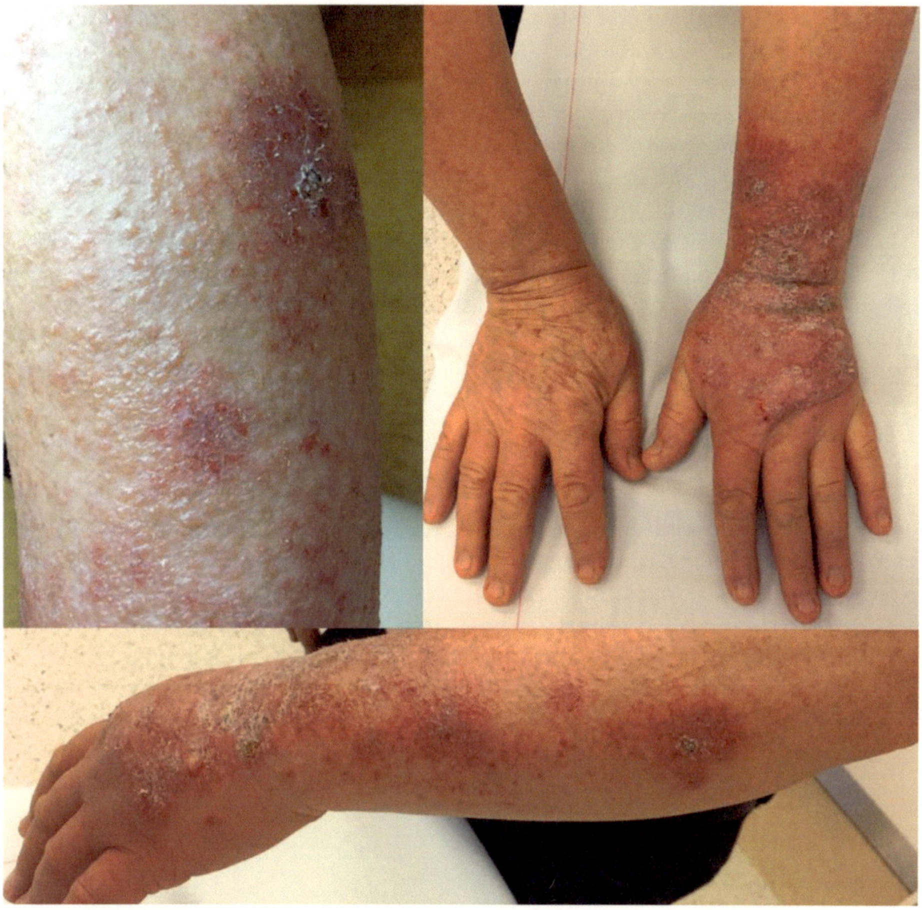

**Figure 3.**
*Irritative contact dermatitis is caused by 5% 5-FU cream, when applied to more areas than recommended.*

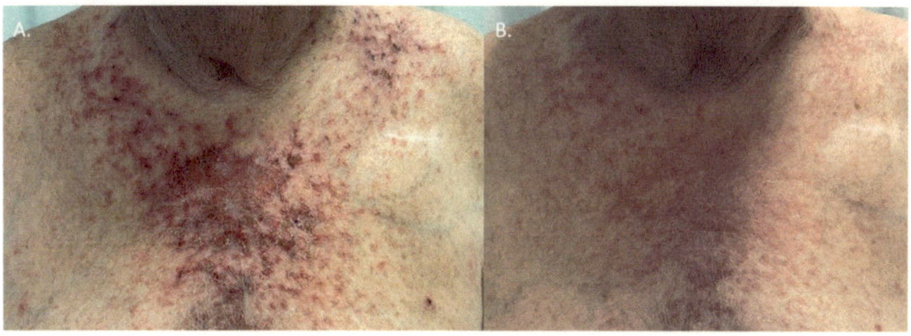


**Figure 4.**
*Irritative contact dermatitis by 5% 5-FU cream (A), and 2 weeks after application of topical steroid (B).*

side effects are hyperpigmentation, hypopigmentation, onycholysis, photosensitivity, and telangiectasia. If the erosions become superinfected, secondary bacterial infections can occur. Applying it on the face can trigger the reactivation of previous diseases, such as herpes simplex virus, rosacea, or seborrheic dermatitis [51].

More severe topical adverse events can be allergic contact dermatitis, with redness, swelling, papulation, vesiculation, oozing and weeping, and even blistering [52].

Extreme inflammatory skin reaction has been reported when it is applied under wraps, which increases the contact time and penetration of 5-FU into the skin [53].

A life-threatening case of toxicity has been reported after topical 5% 5-FU by Johnson in 1999 [54], and one with the lower-strength 0.5% 5-FU [55]. Both of these patients suffered from dihydropyrimidine dehydrogenase deficiency.

In the management of the side effects, the first step is the withdrawal of the 5-FU. Analgesics, moisturizers, and if there are severe erosions appropriate dressing can be given to the patients, in the case of superinfection antibiotics should be introduced. In severe irritant or allergic contact dermatitis topical steroids may be administered.

### *3.1.7 Administration of 5-fluorouracil*

The adequate application of 5% 5-FU results in maximum efficacy and minimal side effects. Before applying the cream, the area to be treated should be washed with water and dried. Afterward the cream is applied thinly with a cotton ball or with the tip of the finger. If no gloves are worn, the hands should be washed immediately.

The cream should cover the area to be treated and can go max 2–3 mm beyond the visible border of the lesion. The area to be treated at a time cannot exceed 23 cm × 23 cm. Larger areas should be treated one section at a time. The cream should be used twice daily for 3–4 weeks, but this may be extended until there is a marked inflammatory response, preferably with some erosions. Exposure to UV radiation (e.g., natural sunlight, tanning salon) should be avoided.

## 4. Conclusions

Even though surgical treatment is the first choice of care for BCCs, 5-fluorouracil cream in 5% concentration is a good treatment option for sBCCs in certain circumstances. These include patients who wish to avoid procedures or are not good surgical candidates or have many sBCCs. Disadvantages of topical therapy are the lack of histological control and the relatively limited depth of action, therefore 5-FU generally is not recommended in other types of BCCs. Although there are some case study series of combination therapies to enhance the penetration of 5-FU, but further studies are needed.

Today, we have only one available study on long-term follow-up, where the tumor-free survival rate was 70% at 5 years. Comparing the efficacy of 5% 5-FU to imiquimod with the same indication, the latter was shown superior. The advantage of 5-FU over imiquimod is that it is less expensive. To choose the appropriate topical agent for the treatment of sBCC, these factors and patients' preferences should be taken into account.

## Acknowledgements

The research was financed by the Thematic Excellence Program 2021 Health Subprogramme of the Ministry for Innovation and Technology in Hungary, within the framework of the EGA-10 project of the University of Pécs.

## Conflict of interest

The authors declare no conflict of interest.

## Author details

Csongor Németh, Rolland Gyulai and Zsuzsanna Lengyel*
Department of Dermatology, Venerology and Oncodermatology, University of Pécs, Pécs, Hungary

*Address all correspondence to: lengyel.zsuzsanna@pte.hu

## References


[1] Ramelyte E, Nägeli MC, Hunger R, et al. Swiss recommendations for cutaneous basal cell carcinoma. Dermatology. 2023;**239**(1):122-131. DOI: 10.1159/000526478

[2] NCCN Guidelines Version 2.2022. Basal Cell Skin Cancer

[3] Peris K, Fargnoli MC, Garbe C, et al. Diagnosis and treatment of basal cell carcinoma: European consensus-based interdisciplinary guidelines. European Journal of Cancer. 2019;**118**:10-34. DOI: 10.1016/j.ejca.2019.06.003

[4] Scrivener Y, Grosshans E, Cribier B. Variations of basal cell carcinomas according to gender, age, location and histopathological subtype. The British Journal of Dermatology. 2002;**147**:41-47. DOI: 10.1046/j.1365-2133.2002.04804.x

[5] McCormack CJ, Kelly JW, Dorevitch AP. Differences in age and body site distribution of the histological subtypes of basal cell carcinoma. A possible indicator of differing causes. Archives of Dermatology. 1997;**133**:593-596

[6] Marzuka AG, Book SE. Basal cell carcinoma: Pathogenesis, epidemiology, clinical features, diagnosis, histopathology, and management. The Yale Journal of Biology and Medicine. 2015;**88**:167-179

[7] Reiter O, Mimouni I, Dusza S, et al. Dermoscopic features of basal cell carcinoma and its subtypes: A systematic review. Journal of the American Academy of Dermatology. 2021;**85**:653-664. DOI: 10.1016/j.jaad.2019.11.008

[8] Novartis Pharmaceuticals. To Evaluate the Safety, Local Tolerability, PK and PD of LDE225 on Sporadic Superficial and Nodular Skin Basal Cell Carcinomas (sBCC). ClinicalTrials.gov. 2015. Available from: https://clinicaltrials.gov/ct2/show/record/NCT01033019?term=LDE225&rank=24 [Accessed: February 10, 2023]

[9] Tang T, Tang JY, Li D, et al. Targeting superficial or nodular basal cell carcinoma with topically formulated small molecule inhibitor of smoothened. Clinical Cancer Research. 2011;**17**:3378-3387. DOI: 10.1158/1078-0432.CCR-10-3370

[10] Cosio T, Di Prete M, Di Raimondo C, et al. Patidegib in dermatology: A current review. International Journal of Molecular Sciences. 2021;**22**:10725. DOI: 10.3390/ijms221910725

[11] Kilgour JM, Shah A, Urman NM, et al. Phase II open-label, single-arm trial to investigate the efficacy and safety of topical remetinostat gel in patients with basal cell carcinoma. Clinical Cancer Research. 2021;**27**:4717-4725. DOI: 10.1158/1078-0432.CCR-21-0560

[12] Chen OM, Kim K, Steele C, et al. Advances in management and therapeutics of cutaneous basal cell carcinoma. Cancers (Basel). 2022;**14**:3720. DOI: 10.3390/cancers14153720

[13] Mahatma G, Sweeney AR, Yen MT. Imiquimod for superficial basal cell carcinomas. International Ophthalmology Clinics. 2020;**60**:3-11. DOI: 10.1097/IIO.0000000000000299

[14] Available from: https://www.accessdata.fda.gov/drugsatfda_docs/label/2010/020723s022lbl.pdf [Accessed: February 10, 2023]

[15] Quirk C, Gebauer K, De'Ambrosis B, Slade HB, Meng TC. Sustained clearance of superficial basal cell carcinomas treated with imiquimod cream 5%: Results of a prospective 5-year study. Cutis. 2010;**85**:318-324

[16] Arits AH, Mosterd K, Essers BA, et al. Photodynamic therapy versus topical imiquimod versus topical fluorouracil for treatment of superficial basal-cell carcinoma: A single blind, non-inferiority, randomised controlled trial. The Lancet Oncology. 2013;**14**:647-654. DOI: 10.1016/S1470-2045(13)70143-8

[17] Searle T, Al-Niaimi F, Ali FR. 5-fluorouracil in dermatology: The diverse uses beyond malignant and premalignant skin disease. Dermatologic Surgery. 2021;**47**:e66-e70. DOI: 10.1097/DSS.0000000000002879

[18] Ceilley RI. Mechanisms of action of topical 5-fluorouracil: Review and implications for the treatment of dermatological disorders. The Journal of Dermatological Treatment. 2012;**23**:83-89. DOI: 10.3109/09546634.2010.507704

[19] Ezzedine K, Painchault C, Brignone M. Systematic literature review and network meta-analysis of the efficacy and acceptability of interventions in actinic keratoses. Acta Dermato-Venereologica. 2021;**101**:adv00358. DOI: 10.2340/00015555-3690

[20] Prince GT, Cameron MC, Fathi R, et al. Topical 5-fluorouracil in dermatologic disease. International Journal of Dermatology. 2018;**57**:1259-1264. DOI: 10.1111/ijd.14106

[21] Zhang N, Yin Y, Xu S, et al. 5-fluorouracil: Mechanisms of resistance and reversal strategies. Molecules. 2008;**13**:1551-1569. DOI: 10.3390/molecules13081551

[22] Longley DB, Harkin DP, Johnston PG. 5-Fluorouracil: Mechanisms of action and clinical strategies. Nature Reviews. Cancer. 2003;**3**:330-338. DOI: 10.1038/nrc1074

[23] Ghoshal K, Jacob ST. Specific inhibition of pre-ribosomal RNA processing in extracts from the lymphosarcoma cells treated with 5-fluorouracil. Cancer Research. 1994;**54**:632-636

[24] McNutt NS, Saenz-Santamaria C, Volkenandt M, et al. Abnormalities of p53 protein expression in cutaneous disorders. Archives of Dermatology. 1994;**130**:225-232

[25] Sachs DL, Kang S, Hammerberg C, et al. Topical fluorouracil for actinic keratoses and photoaging: A clinical and molecular analysis. Archives of Dermatology. 2009;**145**:659-666. DOI: 10.1001/archdermatol.2009.97

[26] 5FU and related substances EMEA-H-A31-1481—Assessment Report27 March 2020 EMA/274404/2020 Pharmacovigilance Risk Assessment Committee (PRAC)

[27] Eaglstein WH, Weinstein GD, FrostP. Fluorouracil: Mechanism of action in human skin and actinic keratoses. I. Effect on DNA synthesis in vivo. Archives of Dermatology. 1970;**101**:132-139. DOI: 10.1001/archderm.1970.04000020002002

[28] Klein E, Stoll HL Jr, Milgrom H, et al. Tumors of the skin V. Local administration of anti-tumor agents to multiple superficial basal cell carcinomas. The Journal of Investigative Dermatology. 1965;**45**:489-495

[29] Litwin MS, Ryan RF, Ichinose H, Reed RR, Kremetz ET. Proceedings: Use of 5 fluorouracil in the topical

therapy of skin cancer: A review of 157 patients. Proceedings. National Cancer Conference. 1972;7:549-556. DOI: 10.1002/jso.2930380409

[30] Bahner JD, Bordeaux JS. Non-melanoma skin cancers: Photodynamic therapy, cryotherapy, 5-fluorouracil, imiquimod, diclofenac, or what? Facts and controversies. Clinics in Dermatology. 2013;**31**:792-798. DOI: 10.1016/j.clindermatol.2013.08.020

[31] Efudex-40t (fluorouracil topical cream) prescribing information. Costa Mesa (CA): Valeant Pharmaceuticals International; 2004. Available from: https://www.accessdata.fda.gov/drugsatfda_docs/label/2005/016831s049lbl.pdf [Accessed: February 25, 2023]

[32] Gross K, Kircik L, Kricorian G. 5% 5-Fluorouracil cream for the treatment of small superficial Basal cell carcinoma: Efficacy, tolerability, cosmetic outcome, and patient satisfaction. Dermatologic Surgery. 2007;**33**:433-439. DOI: 10.1111/j.1524-4725.2007.33090.x

[33] Lecluse LL, Spuls PI. Photodynamic therapy versus topical imiquimod versus topical fluorouracil for treatment of superficial basal-cell carcinoma: A single blind, non-inferiority, randomised controlled trial: A critical appraisal. The British Journal of Dermatology. 2015;**172**:8-10. DOI: 10.1111/bjd.13460

[34] Jansen MHE, Mosterd K, Arits AHMM, et al. Five-year results of a randomized controlled trial comparing effectiveness of photodynamic therapy, topical imiquimod, and topical 5-fluorouracil in patients with superficial basal cell carcinoma. The Journal of Investigative Dermatology. 2018;**138**:527-533. DOI: 10.1016/j.jid.2017.09.033

[35] Neale H, Michelon M, Jacob S, et al. Topical 5% 5-fluorouracil versus procedural modalities for squamous cell carcinoma in situ and superficial basal cell carcinoma: A retrospective cohort analysis. Journal of the American Academy of Dermatology. 2022;**87**:423-425. DOI: 10.1016/j.jaad.2021.08.045

[36] Goon PK, Clegg R, Yong AS, et al. 5-fluorouracil "chemowraps" in the treatment of multiple actinic keratoses: A Norwich experience. Dermatologic Therapy. 2015;**5**:201-205. DOI: 10.7759/cureus.15148

[37] Cadinoiu AN, Rata DM, Atanase LI, et al. Formulations based on drug loaded aptamer-conjugated liposomes as a viable strategy for the topical treatment of basal cell carcinoma-in vitro tests. Pharmaceutics. 2021;**13**:866. DOI: 10.3390/pharmaceutics13060866

[38] Kumar S, Sinha VR. Design, development and characterization of topical microemulsions of 5-fluorouracil for the treatment of non melanoma skin cancer and its precursor lesions. Anti-Cancer Agents in Medicinal Chemistry. 2015;**16**:259-268. DOI: 10.2174/1871520615666150907093551

[39] Naguib YW, Kumar A, Cui Z. The effect of microneedles on the skin permeability and antitumor activity of topical 5-fluorouracil. Acta Pharmaceutica Sinica B. 2014;**4**:94-99. DOI: 10.1016/j.apsb.2013.12.013

[40] Fang JY, Hung CF, Fang YP, et al. Transdermal iontophoresis of 5-fluorouracil combined with electroporation and laser treatment. International Journal of Pharmaceutics. 2004;**270**:241-249. DOI: 10.1016/j.ijpharm.2003.10.025

[41] Nguyen BT, Gan SD, Konnikov N, et al. Treatment of superficial basal cell carcinoma and squamous cell carcinoma in situ on the trunk and extremities with ablative fractional laser-assisted delivery of topical fluorouracil. Journal of the

American Academy of Dermatology. 2015;**72**:558-560. DOI: 10.1016/j.jaad.2014.11.033

[42] Fredman G, Wenande E, Hendel K, et al. Efficacy and safety of laser-assisted combination chemotherapy: A follow-up study of treatment with 5-fluorouracil and cisplatin for basal cell carcinoma. Lasers in Surgery and Medicine. 2022;**54**:113-120. DOI: 10.1002/lsm.23497

[43] Soong LC, Keeling CP. Cryosurgery + 5% 5-fluorouracil for treatment of superficial basal cell carcinoma and bowen's disease [formula: See text]. Journal of Cutaneous Medicine and Surgery. 2018;**22**:400-404. DOI: 10.1177/1203475418758973

[44] Diluvio L, Lanna C, Lozzi F, et al. Basal cell carcinomas treated with 0.5% 5-fluorouracil and 10% salicylic acid topical solution. Dermatologic Therapy. 2019;**32**:e12908. DOI: 10.1111/dth.12908

[45] Dillaha CJ, Jansen GT, Honeycutt WM, et al. Further studies with topical 5-fluorouracil. Archives of Dermatology. 1965;**92**:410-417

[46] Efudix (R) [package insert]. Bishops Stortford, UK: Meda Pharmaceuticals Ltd; 2015. Available from: https://www.medicines.org.uk/emc/files/pil.9260.pdf [Accessed: February 27, 2023]

[47] Erlanger M, Martz G, Ott F, et al. Cutaneous absorption and urinary excretion of 6-14C-5-fluorouracil ointment applicated in an ointment to healthy and diseased human skin. Dermatologica. 1970;**140**:7-14. DOI: 10.1159/000252588

[48] Levy S, Furst K, Chern W. A pharmacokinetic evaluation of 0.5% and 5% fluorouracil topical cream in patients with actinic keratosis. Clinical Therapeutics. 2001;**23**:908-920. DOI: 10.1016/s0149-2918(01)80078-3

[49] Rajinikanth P, Chellian J. Development and evaluation of nanostructured lipid carrier-based hydrogel for topical delivery of 5-fluorouracil. International Journal of Nanomedicine. 2016;**11**:5067-5077. DOI: 10.2147/IJN.S117511

[50] Dean L, Kane M, Pratt VM, et al. Fluorouracil Therapy and DPYD Genotype. In: Medical Genetics Summaries Medical Genetics Summaries [Internet]. Bethesda (MD): National Center for Biotechnology Information (US); 2012

[51] Werbel T, Cohen PR. Topical application of 5-fluorouracil associated with distant seborrheic dermatitis-like eruption: Case report and review of seborrheic dermatitis cutaneous reactions after systemic or topical treatment with 5-fluorouracil. Dermatologic Therapy. 2018;**8**:495-501. DOI: 10.1007/s13555-018-0253-2

[52] Farrar CW, Bell HK, King CM. Allergic contact dermatitis from propylene glycol in Efudix cream. Contact Dermatitis. 2003;**48**:345. DOI: 10.1034/j.1600-0536.2003.00143.x

[53] Loyal J, Romano M, Pierson JC. Exuberant inflammatory reaction to occlusion of topical 5-fluorouracil (FU) under a continuous positive airway pressure (CPAP) mask: A warning to dermatologists and patients. JAAD Case Reports. 2016;**2**:278-280. DOI: 10.1016/j.jdcr.2016.05.011

[54] Johnson M, Hageboutros A, Wang K, et al. Life-threatening toxicity in a dihydropyrimidine dehydrogenase—Deficient patient after treatment with topical 5-fluorouracil. Clinical Cancer Research. 1999;**5**:2006-2011

[55] Kishi P, Price CJ. Life-threatening reaction with topical 5-fluorouracil. Drug Safety—Case Reports. 2018;**5**:4. DOI: 10.1007/s40800-017-0068-6

Section 4

# Future Perspectives

Chapter 7

# Perspective Chapter: Imaging of Biological Activity as a Novel Diagnostic Test for Early Melanoma Detection

*Yoav Litvin, Anne Callahan and Catherine Shachaf*


## Abstract

Clinical melanoma identification relies on subjective visual criteria like color, shape, and size. Current imaging technologies rely on similar parameters without insight into underlying biological changes, necessitating invasive diagnostic approaches. Diagnosing lesions that fall into the "grey area," neither clearly melanoma nor benign/common nevi, presents a particular challenge. Stromal tissue remodeling, pivotal in the early stages of malignancy, is intricately linked to integrins, with αvβ3 integrin playing a prominent role and facilitating neoangiogenesis. For this reason, *in vivo* molecular skin fluorescent imaging (mSFI) is a promising solution, providing molecular insights at the point of care for improved patient management. This chapter delves into melanoma development and detection, focusing on the molecular processes in melanocytic lesion transition to malignancy. *In vivo* fluorescence imaging, such as mSFI, can help dermatologists make strategic biopsy decisions by revealing integrin expression in remodeled stroma, shedding light on oncogenic processes.


**Keywords:** melanoma, imaging, integrin, diagnosis, nevi, dysplastic, mSFI

## 1. Introduction

During embryogenesis, melanocytes, which are derived from neural crest cells, migrate throughout the embryo and colonize eyes, skin, and other tissues [1, 2]. In mature skin, melanocytes populate the basal layer of the epidermis, where they produce melanin. The melanin travels to the outer surface of the skin, protecting genetic material in keratinocytes from mutagenic ultraviolet (UV) rays. When the process is perturbed, melanocytes can aggregate and form benign/common nevi (CN), dysplastic nevi (DN), or melanoma, a malignant melanocyte neoplasm. In melanoma, melanocytes undergo transformation into malignant cells, proliferating within the dermis and potentially disseminating via the lymphatic system or bloodstream.

Current scientific consensus suggests a trajectory for the evolution of nevi into melanoma which entails sequential stages, including DN progressing to melanoma *in-situ* (MIS), advancing through the radial growth phase (RGP) to the vertical growth phase (VGP) and culminating in metastatic melanoma. However, not all DN transition to melanoma, as their transformation depends on molecular pathways and genetic signatures which also promote surrounding tissue remodeling. It is still uncertain whether melanoma arises independently or evolves from existing nevi. Technological limitations hinder the ability to track the transition of nevi to MIS/ melanoma, further complicating our understanding of melanoma development. Additionally, once developed, melanomas can outgrow adjacent CN or DN due to their aggressive expansion and tissue remodeling capabilities.

## 2. Genetics and development of nevi and melanoma

Melanoma development entails genetic changes [3] which drive histological alterations within nevi and/or the surrounding microenvironment. The formation of CN has been linked to mutations in the mitogen-activated protein kinase (MAPK) pathway [4], specifically *BRAF*$^{V600E}$ [5, 6]. CN can subsequently undergo limited proliferation and enter a "senescence-like" state [7]. Consequently, most CN do not change in size, likely due to cell cycle arrest, involvement of the immune system and programmed cell death (apoptosis) [8–10]. DN are known as intermediate neoplasms because their atypical histopathology features are not sufficient to be characterized as overt melanoma [11]. They contain a high prevalence of mutations in *NRAS, BRAF*$^{nonV600E}$, *TERT* promoter, and hemizygous alterations of *CDKN2A* (**Figure 1**) [5].

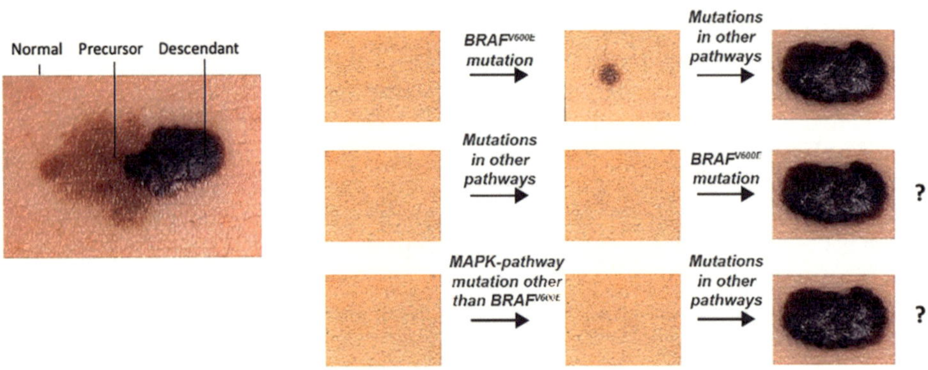


**Figure 1.**
*Possible genetic mutations leading to disparate melanoma trajectories (adapted with permission from [5, 12]).*

Gene expression meta-analyses demonstrate significant overlap of 53 genes in DN and melanoma, supporting the idea that DN can serve as an intermediate phase to MIS. In a recent study [13], up-regulated genes were examined in three RNAseq [12, 14, 15] and four microarray [16–19] studies. Pathways linked to melanoma development were assessed in tissue originating from CN, DN, as well as early stages of melanoma, with the aim of elucidating the trajectories of melanoma development. These analyses revealed the following: (i) several genetic pathways are associated with ongoing structural tissue remodeling and immune response. A gene expression pattern seen with the transition from CN to early-stage melanoma involved alterations in various factors, including matrix metalloproteinases (MMP), cancer-associated fibroblasts (CAFs), chemokines, collagen, ECM genes, laminin, and integrins.

Integrins are recognized for their critical function as adhesion receptors that facilitate tumor proliferation, neoangiogenesis and metastasis [20–24]; (ii) DN may constitute an intermediary stage between CN and early melanoma. Fifty-three genes overlap in DN and melanoma, further substantiating the notion DN can serve as a transitional phase to MIS [5]; (iii) CN in normal skin and CN adjacent to melanoma (AN) are distinct tissue groups with different gene expression profiles. Multiple gene clusters associated with tissue remodeling were identified in AN samples [12, 15] rather than CN [14], including MMP, CAFs, chemokines, collagen, extra-cellular matrix (ECM) genes, laminin, and integrins (see **Figure 2**).

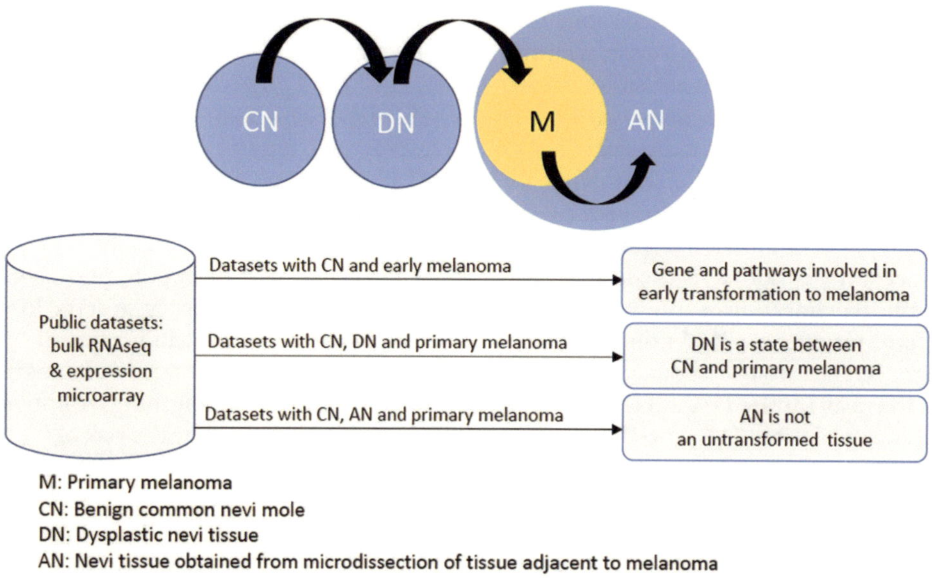


**Figure 2.**
*Summary of molecular signatures [13] that differentiate between CN and early-stage melanomas, implicating up-regulated gene sets and pathways at the earliest stage of melanoma development. A gene profiling comparison of CN and nevi tissue adjunct to melanoma (adjacent nevi (AN)) with melanoma tissue was also performed.*

Studies show only ~30% of melanomas are identified in association with benign nevi tissue, suggesting the majority arise *de novo* [25, 26]. An alternative explanation posits melanoma, due to its aggressive nature, invades by destructively surrounding nevi, eliminating evidence of the originating source tissue at the time of diagnosis. Once developed, all melanomas invade surrounding tissue, including adjacent CN or DN, often obscuring their origins. Because of this, the trajectory of melanoma (whether it originates in existing nevi or develops *de novo*) remains contentious due to lack of technologies able to identify the stage of development and track the low rate of transition of nevi (CN or DN) to MIS. Thus, proper visualization of structural remodeling surrounding nevi may serve to accurately assess nevi with cancerous potential.

## 3. Current diagnostic practices and technologies

Melanoma diagnosis predominantly relies clinically on subjective visual examination of moles on the skin using the ABCDE (Asymmetry, Border, Color, Diameter and Evolving) criteria [27, 28], with dermoscopy improving sensitivity and specificity of clinical assessment [29]. However, visual assessment and dermoscopy are not always sufficient to distinguish between CN and DN, or to adequately assess DN with the potential of developing into melanoma, leading to inconsistent diagnosis and treatment [30]. Moreover, given the potentially fatal nature of melanoma and the prevalence of malpractice lawsuits, physicians often adopt a cautious approach ("when in doubt, cut it out"), opting to excise nevi with a low suspicion of malignancy to mitigate the risk of overlooking cancer. Consequently, numerous benign lesions are needlessly removed. These procedures can be painful and cause infection and scarring. In one study, 940 nevi were clinically evaluated by five dermatologists and then examined by a dermatopathologist who was blinded to prior assessments [31]. Results indicated it was difficult to visually diagnose DN or to gauge the presence or level of dysplasia in nevi during a typical clinical examination.

Several imaging technologies evaluating structural and physical features of nevi have emerged to assist in melanoma diagnosis [32, 33]. These include comparative imaging systems such as reflectance confocal microscopy, total-body photography, and optical coherence tomography (see **Table 1**).

Reflectance confocal microscopy (RCM) is a noninvasive imaging technique used for *in-vivo* examination, offering cellular resolution akin to histological analysis [34]. Since its inception, it has been extensively applied in skin cancer detection, presurgical delineation of tumor boundaries, monitoring treatment efficacy, and tracking tumor recurrence. RCM utilizes a laser as a source of monochromatic and coherent light. Transmittance in Caucasian skin increases progressively with longer wavelengths in the near-infrared region (700–1400 nm), although longer wavelengths offer limited lateral resolution. The power of the laser light source is constrained by the risk of tissue damage and skin sensitivity. The light from these microscopes passes through a beam splitter, a scanning and focusing optical lens, and a skin contact device. This device maintains lateral stability of the skin, reducing motion blurring. It comprises a metal ring and template placed in contact with the patient's skin using double-sided adhesive tape, and it can be magnetically coupled to the microscope housing. It holds the immersion medium, typically water or water-based gels, as their refractive index (1.33) closely matches that of the epidermis (1.34), thus minimizing unnecessary reflection. Within the skin, light is focused on a small tissue spot a few microns in diameter. Reflection occurs at the boundary between cellular structures with different refractive indices, such as membranes, keratohyalin granules, and melanosomes. Reflectance can also arise when the viewed object is similar in size to the illuminating wavelength. By adjusting the depth at which the objective lens focuses in the vertical (z) plane relative to the skin, images of any specific layer within the skin can be captured. This is achieved by scanning horizontally along two orthogonal directions (y and x-axis) parallel to the focal plane and then transmitting these optical signals through the interface software to reconstruct a thin horizontal microscopic image.

Total-body photography (TBP) is presently employed for the surveillance of individuals at high risk for melanoma, used for the potential of earlier melanoma detection [40]. It enables the objective documentation of all existing lesions and the monitoring of changes in these lesions over time. This photography can be accomplished through either 2-dimensional (2D) or 3-dimensional (3D) TBP. In 2D TBP, standard 2D skin images are captured and assembled into a body map, while in 3D TBP, a three-dimensional representation of the patient's surface is generated, sometimes integrated with dermoscopy images. 3D TBP involves capturing numerous overlapping images of the body surface from various perspectives to generate a 3D representation. Unlike traditional 2D TBP, which uses a single camera, 3D TBP utilizes calculated vectors to assign each skin area spatial coordinates in

| Methodologies | Clinical effectiveness | Pros | Cons |
|---|---|---|---|
| Dermoscopy | Sensitivity: 79–93%, specificity: 69–89% | Established technology | Low resolution; shallow penetration depth; additional training required. |
| Total-body photography (TBP) | N/A | Established technology, improved management by clinicians, reduction in patient and physician anxiety. | Large, expensive, complex management and storage, labor-intensive systems. Does not permit monitoring of lesions on genital, acral, and scalp areas, or within body folds. Requires interpretation by trained and experienced personnel. |
| Reflectance confocal microscopy (RCM) | Sensitivity: 92%, specificity: 70%; reduced benign to malignant biopsy ratio in conjunction with dermoscopy. | Superior diagnostic accuracy; cellular-level resolution; high-contrast imaging; strong correlation with histopathology. Absence of artifacts induced by conventional microscopy. In vivo microscopy | Restricted detection range and depth a relatively weak penetration of only ~200 μm in skin, preventing imaging of structures located in the reticular dermis; interpretation of RCM sections difficult due to their orientation, i.e., perpendicular to the conventional vertically oriented histological sections; prolonged acquisition duration; dependence on favorable skin condition; high cost; additional training necessary. |
| Optical coherence tomography (OCT) | N/A | Cross-sectional images of skin with a resolution of a few micrometers, significantly lower than RCM. Assessing OCT images in a vertical orientation facilitates comparison with traditional histological sections. Quick image capture; enhanced depth penetration; vertical imaging capability; vascularization assessment. | Limited resolution (excluding HD-OCT); accuracy in diagnosing malignant melanoma lags behind RCM due to its lower imaging resolution; dependent on favorable skin condition; costly; additional training required. |
| Molecular skin fluorescence imaging (mSFI) | 100% sensitivity, and 95.7% specificity | Easy to use by any trained medical personnel. On site, *in-vivo*, quick results, objective compared to other methodologies. Affordable. Monitors biological activity. | Novel technology, cannot use on acral lesions, tattoos, and breached skin. |

*Source: Adapted from [33–39].*

**Table 1.**
*Non-invasive imaging techniques.*

three dimensions. 3D TBP can greatly assist in lesion localization during follow-up, and both methods can enhance the early detection of melanoma by improving diagnostic accuracy in high-risk patients [41]. Total-body photography offers the benefit of monitoring the patient's entire skin surface rather than just specific individual lesions.

Optical coherence tomography (OCT) is a relatively recent non-invasive optical imaging technique that offers real-time visualization of tissues *in vivo* [42]. It operates on the principle of Michelson interferometry, utilizing infrared radiation to generate high-resolution, 2- or 3-dimensional cross-sectional images of tissue microstructural morphology. OCT delivers depth-resolved images with resolutions down to a few micrometers, and penetration depths of several millimeters. The depths vary according to tissue characteristics. This technique utilizes infrared light to assess the scattering properties of tissues, including echo time delay and the intensity of backscattered or backreflected light. It offers real-time cross-sectional as well as enface sectional images of the subsurface microstructure of tissues with micrometer resolution, allowing visualization of skin morphology such as the epidermis, dermis, dermoepidermal junction, nodular and fibrous structures, cellular elements, hair follicle units, blood vessels and sweat glands, and examination of altered skin architecture in superficial skin lesions. High-definition OCT (HD-OCT) is a technique that builds upon conventional OCT principles by employing parallel time-domain interferometry and adaptive optics.

The technologies detailed above focus on the physical properties of the lesions themselves. The early progression from benign to malignant growth relies on vital support from the ECM and neoangiogenesis, facilitating tumor expansion and connection to the circulatory system [23, 24, 43–45]. Recent findings demonstrate structural remodeling associated with melanoma has an impact on its neighboring environment. When compared with CN surrounded by healthy tissue, AN exhibit indications of structural remodeling, suggesting the potential for malignancy [13]. Consequently, incorporating patients' medical history and current skin condition into nevi diagnostics, regardless of their current melanoma risk based on ABCDE criteria, is crucial. Additionally, early detection of molecular processes indicative of melanoma or nevi with malignant potential can significantly improve patient outcomes [46].

To overcome subjective interpretation, usability challenges, device costs, and lengthy diagnostic processes, a precise, non-invasive, real-time test is urgently needed. Such an approach could revolutionize melanoma diagnosis, facilitating timely interventions and reducing unnecessary biopsies.

## 4. Structural tissue remodeling

Identifying early melanoma evolution and common biomarkers across melanoma types could enhance diagnosis, enabling better recovery, innovative treatments, and minimizing biopsy-related complications like pain, scarring, and infection.

Structural remodeling in the tumor microenvironment has become an emerging target for evaluation and subsequent diagnosis. In the early 1970s, Folkman demonstrated that growth of initiating tumor microfoci was limited by the distance oxygen could diffuse from the nearest capillary blood vessel (<250 micrometers) [47, 48]. Indeed, most melanocytic neoplasms and tumor microfoci arrest at a dormant stage and are harmless unless they recruit new capillaries carrying oxygen and nutrients required for growth [49]. Transition from benign to cancerous growth depends on crucial support from the ECM and neoangiogenesis, which provides the early growth with space and nutrients while connecting the tumor to the circulatory system [43–45]. As progression occurs, melanoma develops an intricate vascular network with tumor cells expressing the laminin receptor, facilitating their attachment to vascular walls. Neoangiogenesis signals a shift from the avascular to the vascular phase of tumor growth, including increased aggressiveness, metastasis, and poorer prognosis [50–52]. The level of angiogenesis observed in human melanoma results from the interplay of multiple angiogenic and antiangiogenic factors synthesized by diverse cell types within the microenvironment of the melanoma.

In addition to nutrients and oxygen, tumors require space and the ability to override the embryonic tissue program determining organ shape and size. Moreover, tumor cells must overcome the body's immune surveillance function which keeps microfoci from growing. *RAS* mutations and UV radiation photodamage may initiate the first stages of melanoma formation. Genetically altered melanocytes secrete cytokines and growth factors, flooding their surrounding macroenvironment. Eventually, the host tissue responds by degrading the surrounding ECM to create space, which allows the emerging melanoma to expand. This process is mediated by CAFs residing within or around the tumor [53]. CAFs upregulate MMPs that degrade ECM proteins such as collagen, fibronectin, elastin, and proteoglycans. MMPs 8, 12, 14, 15, and 16 promote the less aggressive RGP, and MMP 13 promotes the VGP characteristic of more aggressive melanomas [54]. MMPs digest collagen and fibronectins in the ECM, releasing arginine-glycine-aspartic acid (RGD) fragments that bind and activate integrin cell surface receptors [55–57], particularly integrins $\alpha v\beta 3$, $\alpha v\beta 5$ and $\alpha 5\beta 1$ [22], promoting tumor growth, metastasis [21], and neoangiogenesis.

## 5. Integrins

Integrins mediate bidirectional signaling between cells and their environment and play a pivotal role in melanoma progression. Their activation triggers intracellular signal transduction, cell migration, and survival, directly influencing angiogenesis, lymphangiogenesis, and melanoma proliferation [21, 22, 58]. These receptors facilitate the transition of melanoma from RGP to VGP.

Due to its pivotal role in melanoma growth and proliferation, radiolabeled RGD has been used as an imaging tool [59] in melanoma [60] and breast cancer [61] as well as other late-stage solid cancers [62]. In addition, presence of $\beta 3$ integrin has been shown to be associated with sentinel lymph node metastasis of melanoma [63]. Further, Cilengitide (EMD 121974, Merck KGaA, Darmstadt, Germany), a cyclized pentapeptide Arg-Gly-Asp-DPhe-(NMeVal) RGD fragment designed to block integrin-mediated activity found in solid tumors, has been tested as a therapeutic with varying levels of success in: (i) pharmacokinetic studies [64]; (ii) patients with solid tumors [65]; (iii) patients with advanced solid tumors [66]; (iv) children with refractory brain tumors [67]; (v) patients with recurrent malignant glioma [68]; (vi) treatment of head and neck tumors [69]; (vii) second-line treatment for patients with advanced non-small-cell lung cancer [70]; (viii) patients with metastatic melanoma [60]; (ix) advanced unresectable pancreatic cancer [71]; (x) prostate cancer [72]; and (xi) asymptomatic patients with androgen-independent prostate cancer [73], suggesting a crucial role of integrin activity in cancer development.

## 6. Molecular imaging

*In vivo* molecular imaging entails observing, describing, and quantifying biological activities at the molecular and cellular levels within humans and other living organisms [74]. In the realm of molecular imaging, various techniques have been explored, including nuclear magnetic resonance, ultrasound, radiation and optical methods. Among these, two approaches are notable for their sensitivity. Nuclear medical imaging involves administering a radioactive molecular probe into the body, and then tracking its distribution and kinetics through positron emission tomography (PET) and single-photon emission computed tomography (SPECT). This method allows for whole-body imaging due to the unlimited depth penetration of radiation. It also offers quantitative molecular imaging capabilities. In contrast, optical molecular imaging utilizes a fluorescent probe, avoiding exposure to ionizing radiation and offering real-time imaging with high spatial resolution at a lower cost. However, its imaging capabilities are limited to the body surface, precluding whole-body imaging.

In *in vivo* optical imaging, light absorption, scattering, and autofluorescence in biological tissue can compromise quantitative precision and sensitivity. To mitigate these effects, fluorescence probes with emission and excitation wavelengths in the near infrared region (700–900 nm) are essential, as they experience minimal interference from endogenous molecules. Effective fluorescent molecular probes for in vivo imaging must meet several criteria: (i) near-infrared excitation and emission wavelengths with optimal tissue penetration; (ii) efficient delivery to target tissues; (iii) high signal-to-noise ratio for target versus non-target fluorescence intensity; and (iv) excellent safety profile.

## 7. *In vivo* molecular imaging of αvβ3 integrin

Harnessing the potential of imaging could offer a non-invasive method to detect tissue remodeling associated with melanocytic transition, aiding in accurate and early diagnosis paired with personalized treatment strategies.

Radioactive imaging tags are used to image angiogenic tumors, yet optical imaging alternatives are safer (no ionization), have superior sensitivity and are more cost effective and convenient to use [75]. Optical fluorescence imaging may be especially practical for detecting tissue remodeling associated with melanocytic transition, promising a less invasive way to detect pre-cancerous or cancerous tissues [76].

Neto et al. [77] reviewed the importance of αvβ3 integrin expression and signaling in various stages of melanocytic transition. They showed that the highest αvβ3 integrin expression is in MIS and lymph node metastases. Thus, the presence and high expression of αvβ3 integrin in MIS shows promise as a good marker for the earliest stages of melanocytic transition reflective of oncogenic tissue remodeling. A proof-of-concept clinical study [35] geared towards the identification of tissue remodeling associated with αvβ3 integrin expression in nevi demonstrates the utility of this approach. Results can be used to help physicians assess the tissue remodeling activity and neoangiogenesis and decide whether there is emerging melanoma or high potential of the nevus developing into melanoma.

αvβ3 integrin can be imaged using RGD-ligand targeting moieties since it is expressed on tumor blood vessels, yet not on normal tissue vessels [78]. Mono-, di-, and tetrameric RGD peptides conjugated with near infrared fluorescent (NIR) Cy-dyes are commonly utilized for *in vivo* imaging in research [79, 80]. Cyanines, alternatively known as tetramethylindo(di)-carbocyanines, are a synthetic dye family classified within the polymethine group. These studies demonstrate the feasibility of non-invasively detecting and semi-quantifying tumor integrin expression using NIR-fluorescent RGD-conjugated probes administered and analyzed via fluorescent molecular imaging technology. The technology may provide improved specificity and sensitivity for correct diagnosis of skin cancer.

## 8. Molecular skin fluorescence imaging (mSFI)

In a recently published proof-of-concept study [35], Shachaf et al. demonstrated the noninvasive application of *in-vivo* molecular skin fluorescence imaging (mSFI; **Figure 3**), utilizing a fluorescent molecular dye (ORL-1) containing the RGD fragment to image biological tissue remodeling activity in pigmented skin nevi and melanoma. ORL-1's binding in areas surrounding nevi provides valuable information, indicating the presence of premalignant tissue remodeling activity and neoangiogenesis characteristic of melanoma development (**Figure 4**).

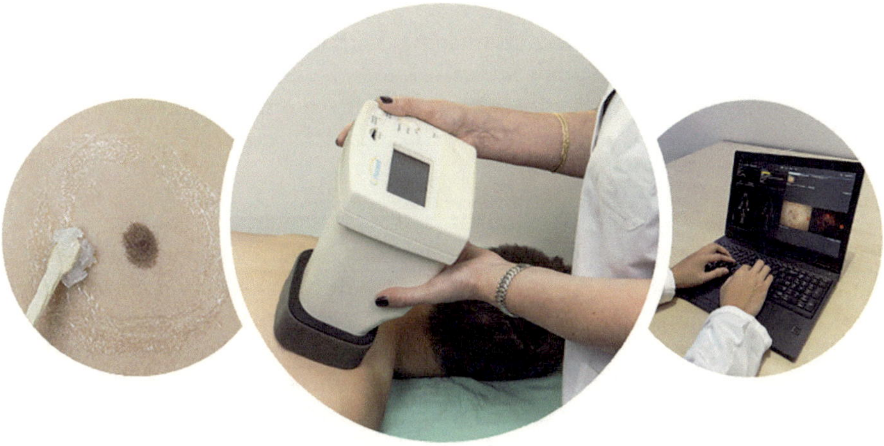

**Figure 3.**
*Molecular skin fluorescence imaging (mSFI) procedure: (i) ORL-1 is topically applied (ii) imager captures white light and fluorescent images; (iii) images are displayed and analyzed using dedicated software.*

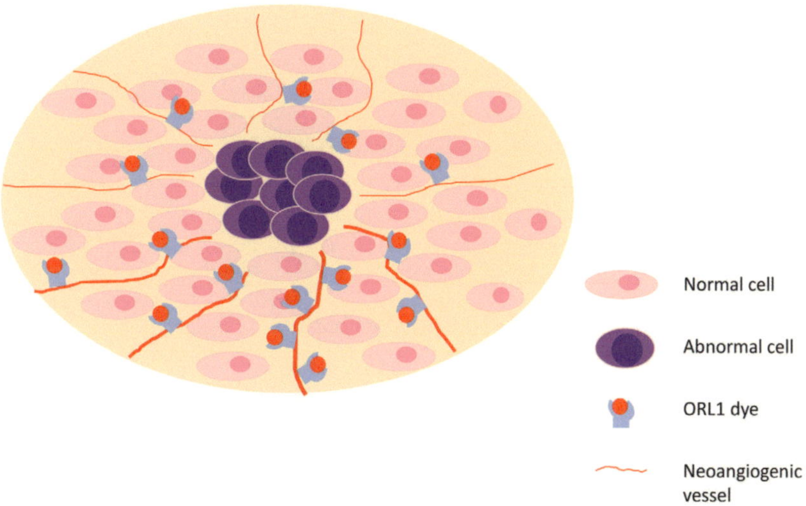


**Figure 4.**
*mSFI imaging captures structural tissue remodeling features associated with melanoma by specifically binding to $\alpha v\beta 3$ integrin receptors (original in Ref. [35]; used with permission).*

Current technologies struggle with early lesion detection due to size or limited cancer cells. mSFI images cellular interactions with the environment, enabling earlier lesion identification than existing methods. Imaging tissue remodeling activity at early stages reduces reliance on subjective or invasive tools like biopsy and reveals biological activity invisible to the naked eye.

Existing technologies struggle to pinpoint lesions in early stages, often due to their small size or limited cancer cell presence. Through cellular imaging and environmental crosstalk analysis, mSFI offers early lesion detection surpassing current methods. This molecular imaging capability addresses a significant clinical need by enabling early detection of structural tissue remodeling activity, reducing reliance on subjective or invasive tools like biopsy while revealing biological activity beyond visible inspection. Utilizing *in vivo* molecular imaging, both melanoma and DN exhibiting similar activity to melanoma can be identified. Identifying integrin and tissue remodeling activity may uncover nevi with potential for melanoma progression.

## 9. Conclusion

This chapter delves into the complexities of melanoma development, the roles of the tumor microenvironment and diagnostic challenges. By acknowledging the subjectivity of current clinical practices, αvβ3 integrin *in vivo* molecular imaging using the innovative technology of mSFI serves as a promising avenue for accurate and early melanoma detection. The integration of αvβ3 integrin analysis into diagnostic protocols could provide clinicians with a more precise and real-time method, overcoming many limitations of current imaging strategies by reducing the need for unnecessary biopsies and offering a valuable tool for personalized treatment strategies. By exploring the intricacies of tissue remodeling associated with melanocytic transition, mSFI offers a non-invasive approach with the potential to revolutionize early detection and improve patient care. Overall, this chapter advocates for a paradigm shift towards objective and advanced diagnostic techniques, with mSFI emerging as a promising methodology for early melanoma detection.

## Conflict of interests

All authors have financial interests in Orlucent, Inc.

## Author details

Yoav Litvin, Anne Callahan and Catherine Shachaf*
Orlucent Inc., United States

*Address all correspondence to: cshachaf@orlucent.com

## References

[1] Mort RL, Jackson IJ, Patton EE. The melanocyte lineage in development and disease. Development. 2015;**142**(4):620-632

[2] Mayor R, Theveneau E. The neural crest. Development. 2013;**140**(11): 2247-2251

[3] Shain AH, Bastian BC. From melanocytes to melanomas. Nature Reviews. Cancer. 2016;**16**(6):345-358

[4] Pollock PM et al. High frequency of BRAF mutations in nevi. Nature Genetics. 2003;**33**(1):19-20

[5] Shain AH et al. The genetic evolution of melanoma from precursor lesions. The New England Journal of Medicine. 2015;**373**(20):1926-1936

[6] Yeh I, von Deimling A, Bastian BC. Clonal BRAF mutations in melanocytic nevi and initiating role of BRAF in melanocytic neoplasia. Journal of the National Cancer Institute. 2013;**105**(12):917-919

[7] Michaloglou C et al. BRAFE600-associated senescence-like cell cycle arrest of human naevi. Nature. 2005;**436**(7051):720-724

[8] Gorgoulis VG et al. Activation of the DNA damage checkpoint and genomic instability in human precancerous lesions. Nature. 2005;**434**(7035):907-913

[9] Campisi J, d'Adda di Fagagna F. Cellular senescence: When bad things happen to good cells. Nature Reviews. Molecular Cell Biology. 2007;**8**(9): 729-740

[10] Kuilman T et al. Oncogene-induced senescence relayed by an interleukin-dependent inflammatory network. Cell. 2008;**133**(6):1019-1031

[11] Duffy K, Grossman D. The dysplastic nevus: From historical perspective to management in the modern era: Part I. Historical, histologic, and clinical aspects. Journal of the American Academy of Dermatology. 2012;**67**(1):1. e1-1.16; quiz 17-8

[12] Shain AH et al. Genomic and transcriptomic analysis reveals incremental disruption of key signaling pathways during melanoma evolution. Cancer Cell. 2018;**34**(1):45-55 e4

[13] Zia A et al. Transcriptome analysis identifies oncogenic tissue remodeling during progression from common nevi to early melanoma. The American Journal of Pathology. Jul 2023;**193**(7):995-1004

[14] Badal B et al. Transcriptional dissection of melanoma identifies a high-risk subtype underlying TP53 family genes and epigenome deregulation. JCI Insight. 2017;**2**(9):1-15

[15] Kunz M et al. RNA-seq analysis identifies different transcriptomic types and developmental trajectories of primary melanomas. Oncogene. 2018;**37**(47):6136-6151

[16] Kabbarah O et al. Integrative genome comparison of primary and metastatic melanomas. PLoS One. 2010;**5**(5):e10770

[17] Mitsui H et al. Discrimination of dysplastic nevi from common melanocytic nevi by cellular and molecular criteria. The Journal of Investigative Dermatology. 2016;**136**(10):2030-2040

[18] Scatolini M et al. Altered molecular pathways in melanocytic lesions.

International Journal of Cancer. 2010;**126**(8):1869-1881

[19] Talantov D et al. Novel genes associated with malignant melanoma but not benign melanocytic lesions. Clinical Cancer Research. 2005;**11**(20):7234-7242

[20] Mason MD, Allman R, Quibell M. Adhesion molecules in melanoma--more than just superglue? Journal of the Royal Society of Medicine. 1996;**89**(7):393-395

[21] Arias-Mejias SM et al. The role of integrins in melanoma: A review. International Journal of Dermatology. 2020;**59**(5):525-534

[22] Huang R, Rofstad EK. Integrins as therapeutic targets in the organ-specific metastasis of human malignant melanoma. Journal of Experimental and Clinical Cancer Research. 2018;**37**(1):92

[23] Kuphal S, Bauer R, Bosserhoff AK. Integrin signaling in malignant melanoma. Cancer Metastasis Reviews. 2005;**24**(2):195-222

[24] Lee JT, Herlyn M. Microenvironmental influences in melanoma progression. Journal of Cellular Biochemistry. 2007;**101**(4):862-872

[25] Lin WM et al. Outcome of patients with de novo versus nevus-associated melanoma. Journal of the American Academy of Dermatology. 2015;**72**(1):54-58

[26] Bevona C et al. Cutaneous melanomas associated with nevi. Archives of Dermatology. 2003;**139**(12):1620-1624; discussion 1624

[27] Friedman RJ et al. The "dysplastic" nevus. Clinics in Dermatology. 2009;**27**(1):103-115

[28] Haenssle HA et al. Results of a surveillance programme for patients at high risk of malignant melanoma using digital and conventional dermoscopy. European Journal of Cancer Prevention. 2004;**13**(2):133-138

[29] Dinnes J et al. Dermoscopy, with and without visual inspection, for diagnosing melanoma in adults. Cochrane Database of Systematic Reviews. 2018;**12**(12):Cd011902

[30] Duffy KL et al. Clinical decision making based on histopathologic grading and margin status of dysplastic nevi. Archives of Dermatology. 2012;**148**(2):259-260

[31] Annessi G et al. Correlation between clinical atypia and histologic dysplasia in acquired melanocytic nevi. Journal of the American Academy of Dermatology. 2001;**45**(1):77-85

[32] Blundo A et al. Comparative analysis of diagnostic techniques for melanoma detection: A systematic review of diagnostic test accuracy studies and meta-analysis. Frontiers in Medicine (Lausanne). 2021;**8**:637069

[33] Meng X et al. Non-invasive optical methods for melanoma diagnosis. Photodiagnosis and Photodynamic Therapy. 2021;**34**:102266

[34] Calzavara-Pinton P et al. Reflectance confocal microscopy for in vivo skin imaging. Photochemistry and Photobiology. 2008;**84**(6):1421-1430

[35] Shachaf A et al. Molecular skin fluorescence imaging: A tool for evaluating early melanoma development. Pigment Cell and Melanoma Research. May 2024;**37**(3):372-377

[36] Dubois A et al. Line-field confocal optical coherence tomography for high-resolution noninvasive imaging of skin tumors. Journal of Biomedical Optics. 2018;**23**(10):1-9

[37] Melanoma Research Alliance—Melanoma Survival Rates. 2022. Available from: https://www.curemelanoma.org/about-melanoma/melanoma-staging/melanoma-survival-rates

[38] Skudalski L et al. Melanoma: How and when to consider clinical diagnostic technologies. Journal of the American Academy of Dermatology. 2022;**86**(3):503-512

[39] Nwaneshiudu A et al. Introduction to confocal microscopy. The Journal of Investigative Dermatology. 2012;**132**(12):e3

[40] Hornung A et al. The value of total body photography for the early detection of melanoma: A systematic review. International Journal of Environmental Research and Public Health. 2021;**18**(4):1-16

[41] Adler NR et al. Methods of melanoma detection and of skin monitoring for individuals at high risk of melanoma: New Australian clinical practice. The Medical Journal of Australia. 2019;**210**(1):41-47

[42] Xiong YQ et al. Optical coherence tomography for the diagnosis of malignant skin tumors: A meta-analysis. Journal of Biomedical Optics. 2018;**23**(2):1-10

[43] Ostrowski SM, Fisher DE. Biology of melanoma. Hematology/Oncology Clinics of North America. 2021;**35**(1):29-56

[44] Croce CM. Oncogenes and cancer. The New England Journal of Medicine. 2008;**358**(5):502-511

[45] Iurlaro R, León-Annicchiarico CL, Muñoz-Pinedo C. Regulation of cancer metabolism by oncogenes and tumor suppressors. Methods in Enzymology. 2014;**542**:59-80

[46] ACS. Key Statistics for Melanoma Skin Cancer. 2022. Available from: https://www.cancer.org/cancer/types/melanoma-skin-cancer/about.html

[47] Cao Y, Langer R. A review of Judah Folkman's remarkable achievements in biomedicine. Proceedings of the National Academy of Sciences of the United States of America. 2008;**105**(36):13203-13205

[48] Folkman J. Tumor angiogenesis: Therapeutic implications. The New England Journal of Medicine. 1971;**285**(21):1182-1186

[49] Folkman J, Kalluri R. Cancer without disease. Nature. 2004;**427**(6977):787

[50] Srivastava A et al. The prognostic significance of tumor vascularity in intermediate-thickness (0.76-4.0 mm thick) skin melanoma. A quantitative histologic study. The American Journal of Pathology. 1988;**133**(2):419-423

[51] Ribatti D, Annese T, Longo V. Angiogenesis and melanoma. Cancers (Basel). 2010;**2**(1):114-132

[52] Kashani-Sabet M et al. Tumor vascularity in the prognostic assessment of primary cutaneous melanoma. Journal of Clinical Oncology. 2002;**20**(7):1826-1831

[53] Nagelkerke A et al. The mechanical microenvironment in cancer: How physics affects tumours. Seminars in Cancer Biology. 2015;**35**:62-70

[54] Pittayapruek P et al. Role of matrix metalloproteinases in photoaging and photocarcinogenesis. International Journal of Molecular Sciences. 2016;**17**(6):1-20

[55] Ruoslahti E. RGD and other recognition sequences for integrins.

Annual Review of Cell and Developmental Biology. 1996;**12**:697-715

[56] Ruoslahti E, Pierschbacher MD. New perspectives in cell adhesion: RGD and integrins. Science. 1987;**238**(4826):491-497

[57] Theocharis AD et al. Extracellular matrix structure. Advanced Drug Delivery Reviews. 2016;**97**:4-27

[58] Avraamides CJ, Garmy-Susini B, Varner JA. Integrins in angiogenesis and lymphangiogenesis. Nature Reviews. Cancer. 2008;**8**(8):604-617

[59] Haubner R. Alphavbeta3-integrin imaging: A new approach to characterise angiogenesis? European Journal of Nuclear Medicine and Molecular Imaging. 2006;**33**(Suppl. 1):54-63

[60] Kim KB et al. A randomized phase II study of cilengitide (EMD 121974) in patients with metastatic melanoma. Melanoma Research. 2012;**22**(4):294-301

[61] Kenny LM et al. Phase I trial of the positron-emitting Arg-Gly-asp (RGD) peptide radioligand 18F-AH111585 in breast cancer patients. Journal of Nuclear Medicine. 2008;**49**(6):879-886

[62] Axelsson R et al. An open-label, multicenter, phase 2a study to assess the feasibility of imaging metastases in late-stage cancer patients with the alpha v beta 3-selective angiogenesis imaging agent 99mTc-NC100692. Acta Radiologica. 2010;**51**(1):40-46

[63] Quattrocchi E et al. β3 integrin immunohistochemistry as a method to predict sentinel lymph node status in patients with primary cutaneous melanoma. International Journal of Dermatology. 2020;**59**(10):1241-1248

[64] Eskens FA et al. Phase I and pharmacokinetic study of continuous twice weekly intravenous administration of cilengitide (EMD 121974), a novel inhibitor of the integrins alphavbeta3 and alphavbeta5 in patients with advanced solid tumours. European Journal of Cancer. 2003;**39**(7):917-926

[65] O'Donnell PH et al. A phase I study of continuous infusion cilengitide in patients with solid tumors. Investigational New Drugs. 2012;**30**(2):604-610

[66] Hariharan S et al. Assessment of the biological and pharmacological effects of the alpha nu beta3 and alpha nu beta5 integrin receptor antagonist, cilengitide (EMD 121974), in patients with advanced solid tumors. Annals of Oncology. 2007;**18**(8):1400-1407

[67] MacDonald TJ et al. Phase I clinical trial of cilengitide in children with refractory brain tumors: Pediatric brain tumor consortium study PBTC-012. Journal of Clinical Oncology. 2008;**26**(6):919-924

[68] Nabors LB et al. Phase I and correlative biology study of cilengitide in patients with recurrent malignant glioma. Journal of Clinical Oncology. 2007;**25**(13):1651-1657

[69] Raguse JD et al. Cilengitide (EMD 121974) arrests the growth of a heavily pretreated highly vascularised head and neck tumour. Oral Oncology. 2004;**40**(2):228-230

[70] Manegold C et al. Randomized phase II study of three doses of the integrin inhibitor cilengitide versus docetaxel as second-line treatment for patients with advanced non-small-cell lung cancer. Investigational New Drugs. 2013;**31**(1):175-182

[71] Friess H et al. A randomized multicenter phase II trial of the angiogenesis inhibitor cilengitide (EMD 121974) and gemcitabine compared with gemcitabine alone in advanced unresectable pancreatic cancer. BMC Cancer. 2006;**6**:285

[72] Alva A et al. Phase II study of cilengitide (EMD 121974, NSC 707544) in patients with non-metastatic castration resistant prostate cancer, NCI-6735. A study by the DOD/PCF prostate cancer clinical trials consortium. Investigational New Drugs. 2012;**30**(2):749-757

[73] Beekman KW et al. Phase II evaluations of cilengitide in asymptomatic patients with androgen-independent prostate cancer: Scientific rationale and study design. Clinical Genitourinary Cancer. 2006;**4**(4):299-302

[74] Saji H. In vivo molecular imaging. Biological and Pharmaceutical Bulletin. 2017;**40**(10):1605-1615

[75] Ye Y, Chen X. Integrin targeting for tumor optical imaging. Theranostics. 2011;**1**:102-126

[76] Tipirneni KE et al. Fluorescence imaging for cancer screening and surveillance. Molecular Imaging and Biology. 2017;**19**(5):645-655

[77] Neto DS et al. Alpha-v-beta3 integrin expression in melanocytic nevi and cutaneous melanoma. Journal of Cutaneous Pathology. 2007;**34**(11):851-856

[78] Danhier F, Le Breton A, Préat V. RGD-based strategies to target alpha(v) beta(3) integrin in cancer therapy and diagnosis. Molecular Pharmaceutics. 2012;**9**(11):2961-2973

[79] Wang F et al. The functions and applications of RGD in tumor therapy and tissue engineering. International Journal of Molecular Sciences. 2013;**14**(7):13447-13462

[80] Wu Y, Cai W, Chen X. Near-infrared fluorescence imaging of tumor integrin alpha v beta 3 expression with Cy7-labeled RGD multimers. Molecular Imaging and Biology. 2006;**8**(4):226-236